CONTEMPORARY ISSUES IN HEAD AND NECK CANCER MANAGEMENT

Edited by **Loredana G. Marcu**

Contemporary Issues in Head and Neck Cancer Management
http://dx.doi.org/10.5772/58653
Edited by Loredana G. Marcu

Contributors

Camile Farah, Jennifer Wu, Keziah John, Loredana G. Marcu, Iuliana Dasu, Alexandru Dasu, Jizhen Lin, Lieping Chen, Jinhuo Lai, Merill Biel, Denise Tostes Oliveira, Federica Ganci, Andrea Sacconi, Valentina Manciocco, Giuseppe Spriano, Giulia Fontemaggi, Giovanni Blandino, Paolo Carlini, Suwarna Dangore-Khasbage

Published by InTech

Janeza Trdine 9, 51000 Rijeka, Croatia

Publishing Process Manager Iva Simcic

Technical Editor InTech DTP team

Cover InTech Design team

First published July, 2015

Printed in Croatia

Additional hard copies can be obtained from orders@intechopen.com

Contemporary Issues in Head and Neck Cancer Management, Edited by Loredana G. Marcu

p. cm.

ISBN 978-953-51-2135-0

For EU product safety concerns:
IN TECH d.o.o., Prolaz Marije Krucifikse Kozulić 3, 51000 Rijeka, Croatia,
info@intechopen.com or visit our website at intechopen.com.

Meet the editor

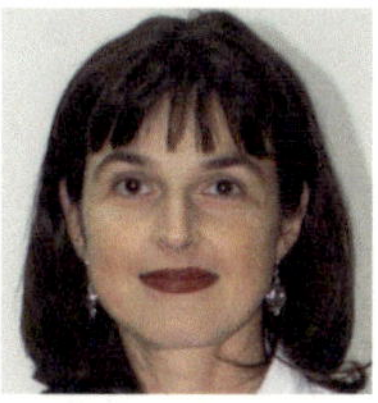

Dr. Loredana Marcu is currently a Professor of Medical Physics at the University of Oradea, Romania and holds affiliation with the University of Adelaide, Australia. She received her PhD in Medical Physics from the University of Adelaide. Her 20 years teaching experience, at both Australian and Romanian universities, has been materialised in seven books published on physics, radiobiology and teaching methodologies, with two more volumes on Medical Physics being currently in press.

She is author of 5 textbooks and university lab guides, and has over 100 publications and conference presentations worldwide. Dr. Marcu is the recipient of the "Boyce Worthley award 2006" given by the Australasian College of Physical Scientists and Engineers in Medicine for her achievements in radiobiology and medical physics.

Contents

Preface

Head and neck cancers comprise of tumours arising in the following anatomical locations: oral cavity, pharynx (nasopharynx, oropharynx, hypopharynx), larynx, paranasal sinuses, nasal cavity and salivary glands. The predominant type consists of squamous cell carcinomas (95%) whilst the remaining are adenocarcinomas or melanomas.

According to the latest Globocan report issued by the International Agency for research on Cancer, the estimated incidence of head and neck cancer (HNC) in 2012 among men represents 7% of all cancers, while in women is 2.6% [1]. While the incidence of head and neck cancers caused by known risk factors such as tobacco smoking and alcohol consumption has lately decreased [2], a relatively new entity of head and neck squamous cell carcinoma, mostly located in the oropharynx was shown to be on the rise and was attributed to the human papillomavirus (HPV) [3]. This distinct entity of head and neck cancer holds different biological characteristics from the non-HPV tumours and responds differently to therapy [3,4]. New treatment challenges are therefore generated that need solutions in the near future.

Conventional treatment techniques such as surgery and radio-chemotherapy have not improved significantly the overall 5-year survival of this disease over the past thirty years. The high mortality rate is due to the fact that most head and neck cancers are diagnosed at advanced stages of the disease. Additionally, given the anatomical location of these tumours, treatment often leads to long-term side effects, which can have a significant impact on the quality of life. Early diagnosis therefore plays a key role in increasing the therapeutic ratio and improving patient survival and quality of life.

As for several other tumour types, radiobiology continues to shape the treatment of head and neck cancers. The original four Rs of radiotherapy (i.e. repair, repopulation, reoxygenation and redistribution along the cell cycle) have been promoted to six Rs by the inclusion of radioresistance and remote effects. New developments related to cancer stem cells and their interaction with the hypoxic environment, as well as the higher radiosensitivity of HPV-positive HNC due to their compromised repair capacity are important elements for new treatment designs.

While the management of head and neck cancer is evolving, there are still several challenges and unanswered questions that need solutions. Further efforts are needed to resolve clinical concerns such as:

• Tumour repopulation during treatment and the role of cancer stem cells in head and neck tumour recurrence;

• Quantitative assessment of radiobiological hypoxia in head and neck tumours and methods to overcome hypoxia-driven radioresistance;

- Treatment individualisation based on tumour kinetics and dynamics;
- Distant metastases and systemic treatment approaches;
- The role of targeted therapy in head and neck cancer;
- Treatment directions for HPV positive oropharyngeal cancer and dose de-escalation;
- Reduction of treatment-related normal tissue complications.

Contemporary Issues in Head and Neck Cancer Management is a small compilation of some topical aspects regarding head and neck cancer treatment, including the etiology of HPV-positive oropharyngeal cancers and risk factors in the young population, the challenge of surgical margin definition and the perennial problem of systemic treatment due to distant metastases. Radiobiological aspects are also covered through the "Rs" of radiotherapy, with a couple of chapters being dedicated to radioresistance and tumour microenvironment. This book comes as an addition to the existing literature that aims to tackle this radiobiologically challenging tumour.

I would like to thank all authors for their hard work and great contributions to this volume of ***Contemporary Issues in Head and Neck Cancer Management***

Prof. Loredana G. Marcu
Faculty of Science, University of Oradea, Romania
School of Chemistry and Physics, University of Adelaide, SA, Australia

References

[1] Ferlay J, Soerjomataram I, Ervik M, Dikshit R, Eser S, Mathers C, et al. GLOBOCAN 2012 v1.0, Cancer Incidence and Mortality Worldwide: IARC CancerBase No. 11, 2013, Lyon, France: International Agency for Research on Cancer. Available from http://globocan.iarc.fr.

[2] Chaturvedi AK, Engels EA, Anderson WF, Gillison ML. Incidence trends for human papillomavirus-related and -unrelated oral squamous cell carcinomas in the United States. J Clin Oncol 2008;26(4):612-9.

[3] Ang KK, Sturgis EM. Human papillomavirus as a marker of the natural history and response to therapy of head and neck squamous cell carcinoma. Semin Radiat Oncol 2012;22(2):128-42.

[4] Urban D, Corry J, Rischin D. What is the best treatment for patients with human papillomavirus-positive and –negative oropharyngeal cancer? Cancer 2014;120(10):1462-70.

Section 1

Radiobiology and Tumour Microenvironment

Chapter 1

Radioresistance in Head and Neck Squamous Cell Carcinoma — Possible Molecular Markers for Local Recurrence and New Putative Therapeutic Strategies

Federica Ganci, Andrea Sacconi,
Valentina Manciocco, Giuseppe Spriano,
Giulia Fontemaggi, Paolo Carlini and
Giovanni Blandino

Additional information is available at the end of the chapter

http://dx.doi.org/10.5772/60081

1. Introduction

Head and neck squamous cell carcinoma (HNSCC) comprises 5.5% of all incidence cancers and is the sixth leading cancer worldwide with approximately 600,000 cases reported annually [1, 2]. The vast majority of them are squamous cell carcinomas that originate in the epithelium of the oral cavity, pharynx and larynx. There is a higher incidence rate in males compared to females and the median age of patients with HNSCC is about 60 years [3]. The main risk factors for HNSCC are tobacco smoking and heavy use of alcohol. In particular, alcohol consumption and tobacco smoking have a synergic effect [4]. The contribution of tobacco exposure to HNSCC carcinogenesis is strongly correlated with the time and rate of the person who smokes and has showed to have site-specific differences according to the anatomical regions, with an increase in sensitivity from the oral cavity down to the larynx [5]. In addition, high-risk infection types of human papillomavirus (especially HPV-16 and 18) is emerging as a major cause of a subgroup of HNSCC, particularly those of the oropharynx and oral cavity [2, 6]. The traditional risk factors, tobacco and alcohol use, do not appear to play a contributing role in HPV-positive cancers [7]. However, it is known that HPV-positive and negative tumors have different clinical, pathological and molecular characteristics and that HPV-positive tumors are associated with a more favorable outcome [2, 6] and better response to standard therapy.

Many molecular studies show that these HNSCC may not be as homogeneous as previously supposed. This indicates the need to obtain a more detailed molecular characterization in order to stratify patients better. This ultimately is likely to provide a more rational therapeutic approach, potentially relevant to diagnosis and prognosis of this poorly defined subset of HNSCC cancer.

2. Therapy strategies and molecular mechanisms of radioresistance

HNSCC is typically characterized by locoregional diffusion and low propensity to develop distant metastasis. Due to the lack of symptoms in the early stage of the disease, about two thirds of patients are diagnosed in advanced stage with lymph node metastases. Local recurrence affects about 50-60% of patients and metastases develop in 15-20% of cases [8], with the five-year overall survival rate less than 50% [8, 9]. Locoregional failure is the most common cause of death in patients affected by HNSCC [10]. Recurrence may arise from residual neoplastic cells that survive to the treatment or from underlying field cancerization. Indeed, one key feature of HNSCC is the insurgence of recurrences after seemingly complete surgical resection, probably due to the existence of preneoplastic processes at multiple sites in the mucosa ("field cancerization" hypothesis). These preneoplastic tissues are apparently tumor-free when analyzed at histological level but present several genetic alterations when analyzed at a molecular level [11, 12].

Typically, HNSCC treatment consists of surgical resection followed by ionizing radiation or chemoradiation, or chemoradiation alone. Therapeutic strategy choice depends on disease stage: tumors at early stage are treated with surgery or radiotherapy. Surgery can be performed if complete tumor excision is possible and radiation can be used postoperatively when surgical margins are positive for the presence of tumor cells and/or if lymphovascular invasion by tumor is found. Platinum-based agents, in particular cisplatin (CDDP), are the conventional chemotherapeutic drugs for HNSCC treatment. More advanced cancers require multimodality therapy combining surgery, radiation and chemotherapy. Concurrent chemoradiation is the preferred treatment for advanced inoperable HNSCC [13-15]. These standard therapies have some limitations; they have several side effects and generally more than 50% of HNSCC patients relapse. The toxicities are mainly due to non-selective nature of treatment. However, resistance to chemoradiotherapy frequently occurs and is associated with poor outcome. This is the major clinical problem in HNSCC patients and relies on the fact that recurrence is often related to an intrinsic tumor radioresistance [14].

Molecular mechanisms underlying the resistance to radiotherapy or combined treatments mainly involve intracellular pathways related to cell proliferation, apoptosis, DNA repair and angiogenesis [13, 14, 16, 17]. To date, the main molecular mechanisms for radioresistance are:

- The hypoxia phenomenon
- Alterations in the Epidermal Growth Factor Receptor (EGFR)- PI3K/Akt pathway
- Epithelial Mesenchymal Transition (EMT) process

- The deregulation in p53 signaling cascades
- Alterations in the expression of angiogenic factors
- The presence of cancer stem cells (CSCs) subpopulation in tumor tissue

2.1. Hypoxia

Hypoxia is a common phenomenon present in many tumors and is associated with poor prognosis, malignant transformation and therapy resistance [18, 19]. In solid tumors, including HNSCC, oxygen is frequently reduced as the result of intermittent blood flow arising from the abnormal tumor microvasculature. Under oxygen deficiency, hypoxic tumor cells can activate the expression of hypoxia-inducible genes, functionally related to pro-survival, anti-apoptosis, angiogenesis, DNA-repair and metabolism signaling pathways [18, 20]. In particular, tumor cells switch their glucose metabolism from the oxygen-dependent tricarboxylic acid (TCA) cycle to oxygen-independent glycolysis metabolic pathway; as a consequence, hypoxic cells use glycolysis as main mechanism to produce ATP.

A key transcription factor having a central role in hypoxia-related gene expression changes is hypoxia-inducible transcription factor 1 (HIF-1). In normoxia, HIF-1α undergoes rapid hydroxylation and degradation. In hypoxia, hydroxylation is prevented, stabilized HIF-1α binds to HIF-1β and the heterodimer binds to hypoxia response elements in target genes, such as glycolytic enzymes, angiogenic molecules (among which VEGFA), survival and growth factors (among which EGF, PDGF and TGF-β), chaperons and other apoptosis resistance-related proteins [13, 18, 21].

DNA double-stranded breaks (DSB) are the main DNA lesions leading to cell killing after radiotherapy. Oxygen is known to be a potent radiosensitizer and, through interaction with the radicals formed following radiation, it is essential for the promotion of radiation-induced DNA damage. Oxygen deficiency causes a reduction in reactive oxygen species (ROS) production and a deficit in radiation-induced DNA damage [20]. In agreement with these evidences, cells irradiated in the presence of air are about three times more sensitive than cells irradiated under conditions of severe hypoxia [22].

One of the evidences linking hypoxia to radiation response is a correlation between tumor control and hemoglobin levels [23], which is also related to oxygenation of solid tumors. Indeed, high hemoglobin (Hb) level, prior to and during treatment, has been associated with good prognosis in HNSCC patients treated with radiotherapy [23].

Hypoxia problem is particularly relevant in smoker patients. Indeed, in these HNSCC patients, the low oxygen level is also influenced by the formation of carboxyhemoglobin (COHb) and nicotine vase constrictive effect. As a consequence, the response to treatment and survival of smoker patients is significantly reduced compared to nonsmokers [23].

Given the influence of hemoglobin on tumor oxygenation and radiotherapy response, many researches tried to find methods able to increase Hb level in HNSCC patients having low Hb level, prior to and during radiation treatment; transfusion, or erythropoietin stimulating agents, are some of them, but unfortunately did not result in improved outcome or response to therapy [23]. To date, the main radiosensitizing and cytotoxic agents used in the clinical practice for hypoxic cells targeting are nitroimidazoles, which have also been shown to improve locoregional control, when applied in conjunction with radiation [20].

There is also interest in the use of nitroimidazoles as noninvasive hypoxia markers [24, 25]. Indeed, it remains difficult to identify hypoxic tumors and those patients most likely to benefit from hypoxia modification therapy. Under hypoxic conditions, nitroimidazoles are converted into reactive intermediates, which then become covalently bound to macromolecules within the cell. Nitroimidazoles labeling with an appropriate isotope or immunologically recognizable marker allows the bioreduced compound to be detected, indicating the presence of hypoxia.

Additional indirect non-invasive techniques being explored to identify hypoxic tumors include measuring the immunohistochemical expression of hypoxia-regulated proteins, such as carbonic anhydrase 9 (CA9) and HIF-1α [26, 27]. This represents an attractive approach for routine clinical use, but is limited by the variability of expression of these markers within a tumor and by the lack of hypoxia specificity of individual proteins. An attempt to overcome these problems has been carried out by searching for tumor hypoxia gene signatures by meta-analysis of transcriptome datasets [28-30]. Winter and colleagues defined an *in vivo* hypoxia metagene by clustering around the RNA expression of a set of known *in vitro* hypoxia-regulated genes; this signature was also validated as a prognostic factor for recurrence-free-survival in an independent data set [30].

2.2. Alterations in the Epidermal Growth Factor Receptor (EGFR)-PI3K/Akt pathway

Epidermal growth factor receptor (EGFR) is a transmembrane protein with tyrosine kinase activity that is overexpressed in about 90% of HNSCC, even if its expression is highly variable according to different subgroups of head and neck tumors as well as within the same tumor type [2, 14]. Stimulation by extracellular soluble ligands as epidermal growth factor (EGF) and transforming growth factors (TGFs) induces a conformational change leading to receptor heterodimerization with one of its family members (ErbB2, ErbB3, ErbB4); this causes auto-phosphorylation of the receptor intracellular domain and subsequent internalization followed by the activation of multiple signaling pathways, such as Ras-MAPKs (mitogen-activated protein kinases), extracellular signal-regulated kinases (ERKs), phosphatidylinositol-3-kinase-AKT (PI3-K/AKT), signal transducers and activators of transcription (STAT) and phospholipase C gamma (PLC-g) pathways [20].

High EGFR expression correlates with poor prognosis and resistance to conventional radiotherapy. EGFR expression can also be activated by the ionizing radiation itself, leading to increased radioresistance [20]. EGFR activation is also involved in increased proliferation rate and consequent repopulation, rendering radiotherapy ineffective [14].

Key proteins activated by EGFR are AKT and Ras; the first one is a kinase which phosphorylates multiple downstream effectors, stimulating cell survival and inhibiting apoptosis; Ras is a cell membrane protein able to stimulate a tyrosine kinase cascade, including B-RAF, MEK, MAPK proteins, by which Myc, FOS and Jun translocate in the nucleus finally promoting cell proliferation. This cascade is also able to stimulate the production of EGFR monomers, TGFs and amphiregulin (AREG), contributing to paracrine EGFR activation [14]. Other proteins activated by EGFR are cyclin D1 and Pim-1, involved in cell cycle progression and inhibition of apoptosis; for the activation of both, the signal is mediated by STATs proteins [31, 32]. In addition, the interaction between EGFR-PI3-K/AKT and HIF pathways was also observed under hypoxic conditions, providing evidences on the correlation between EGFR signaling and the induction of angiogenic proteins, such as VEGFA, which is a downstream target of HIF-1 [20]

A subgroup of HNSCC (40%) expresses a truncated splicing variant of the EGFR, called EGFRvIII, in which the ligand-binding domain is altered, due to the deletion of amino acids 6-273. This alteration causes a permanent phosphorylation and activation of the receptor, also in the absence of EGF and TGFs ligands binding. As wild-type EGFR, EGFRvIII is implicated in increased cell proliferation, cell survival, motility and invasion. This variant is absent in normal tissues [17].

Besides EGFR overexpression, other mechanisms are involved in PI3K/Akt signaling hyper-activation, such as Ras activation, PI3-K gene mutation, Akt gene amplification and loss of tumor suppressor protein PTEN [14].

2.3. Epithelial Mesenchymal Transition (EMT) process

Another important mechanism by which radiotherapy can fail in HNSCC is epithelial to mesenchymal transition (EMT) process. When EMT occurs, epithelial cells change in mesenchymal phenotype which is characterized by reduction of the matrix contact, cell–cell adhesion followed by an increase in cell migration and motility. A crucial step of EMT is the loss of E-cadherin, a strong epithelial marker involved in adherens junction that anchors epithelial cells to each other [33]. A reduction of E-cadherin level was observed in HNSCC, especially in poorly differentiated tumors. In addition, many studies have demonstrated that aberrant E-cadherin expression is associated with poor outcome and local recurrence in HNSCC [34]. Loss or decrease of E-cadherin expression causes the translocation of β-catenin protein from the cell membrane to the nucleus to induce transcription of EMT-related genes, such as TWIST and SNAIL1 [33]. Another important protein involved in EMT is vimentin, which is an intermediate filament protein used as a marker for mesenchymal cells and is associated with the migratory phenotype, local recurrence and survival in HNSCC [34, 35]. Also fibronectin, a glycoprotein which mediates cellular interaction with extracellular matrix, plays an important role in migration, growth and adhesion of cells; its expression can be promoted by SNAIL and TWIST transcription factors [33]. Fibronectin is expressed at high level in tumors and blood plasma of HNSCC patients and has been proposed as biomarker of poor response to radiotherapy [36].

2.4. *TP53* gene deregulation

TP53 is a tumor suppressor gene, which functions in carcinogenesis by initiating G1 arrest in response to certain DNA damages and apoptosis. About 40-70% of HNSCC has mutation in *TP53* gene, leading to inactivation of its product [37]. Indeed, mutant p53 proteins are unable to transcriptionally regulate wt-p53 target genes and to exert antitumor effects such as apoptosis, growth arrest, differentiation and senescence. On the other hand, countless evidence has demonstrated that at least certain mutant forms of the p53 protein may possess gain of function activity, thereby positively contributing to the development, maintenance and spreading of many types of tumor, including HNSCC [38, 39]. The prognostic role of p53 alteration in HNSCC is controversial. However, generally, deregulation of p53 protein predicts shorter overall survival, local recurrence and cancer treatment failure [40-44].

In particular, p53 alteration leads to an impaired capability to arrest cell cycle and to inhibit apoptosis. In addition, in this condition also DNA damage repair results compromised. As a consequence, tumor cells carrying *TP53* mutation are less sensitive to radiation-induced cell death and are unable to restore DNA integrity, thus accumulating several genetic mutations which lead to increased tumor heterogeneity and finally to resistance to conventional therapy [14].

In addition, several evidences show that its prognostic value depends on the *TP53* protein domain affected by mutation [43-46]. One of the main classifications of *TP53* mutation used in HNSCC is "disruptive" versus "not-disruptive"; any mutation in L2 or L3 loop of the DNA-binding domain resulting in a polarity change of the protein or any stop codon was classified as disruptive [44]. Disruptive *TP53* mutations were associated with poor outcome and increased radioresistance [44, 46]. Other studies have proposed an alternative classification by which mutations in DNA-binding regions, especially in L2 and L3+LSH motifs, were associated with poorer prognosis and clinical response to radiotherapy [45].

Of note, emerging evidences show that senescence may play a role in the radiation response by wild-type p53 [47]. Senescence is a form of cell cycle arrest in which cells lack replicative potential while remaining metabolically active, and was found to correlate with radiosensitivity in HNSCC [46]. In the proposed model, in the presence of *TP53* wild type or nondisruptive mutation, radiation promotes the induction of ROS production and p21 protein expression, which are critical mediators of cellular senescence. *TP53* disruptive mutations cause cellular senescence inhibition by reduction of radiation-induced ROS, thus driving resistance to radiotherapy [46].

2.5. Alterations in the expression of angiogenic factors

Angiogenesis is a process by which new blood vessels grow up from preexisting capillaries. Because expanding tumors have a continuous need for oxygen and nutrients, tumor cells induce angiogenesis. In particular, by secreting a variety of growth factors they activate the endothelial cells, constituting the inner lining of blood vessels, which produce proteases that degrade the basal membrane and extracellular matrix components. As a consequence, the endothelial cells can proliferate and migrate forming new capillary beds. Because in tumors new blood vessels are irregular and disorganized, the oxygen supply inside the tissue is not homogenous, resulting in continuous angiogenesis stimulation [48].

The main actors of this process are vascular endothelial growth factor (VEGF), fibroblast growth factor (FGF) and matrix metalloprotease (MPP) family proteins.

VEGF family consists of seven ligands, which play a central role in the formation of new blood vessels; VEGFA is the best known agent that induces angiogenesis by binding two receptor tyrosine kinases, VEGFR-1 and VEGFR-2. VEGFA is able to promote development of the vascular system, cell migration, survival and induction of MMPs [13]; it also activates PI3K/AKT and Ras/MAPK signaling pathways [49]. There are increasing evidences that angiogenic response of irradiated tumor cells is related with decreasing radiation sensitivity and head and neck cancer progression. In a meta-analysis of 12 studies including 1002 patients affected by cancer of oral cavity, pharynx and larynx, VEGF expression positivity was associated with a two folds higher risk of death at 2 years of follow-up [50].

Release of VEGF and bEGF by epithelial tumor cells after irradiation is a common response mechanism by which cancer cells may survive and become protected from radiation-induced cell death [51]. Therefore, the level of VEGF and bEGF prior to and during treatment may be relevant for successful therapy.

2.6. Cancer Stem Cells (CSCs)

Cancer stem cells (CSCs) have been defined by Clarke et al., as a small tumor subpopulation possessing the capability to self-renewal and causing the heterogeneous lineage of cancer cells inside the tumor [52]. They are functionally defined as a subset of tumor cells with ability of self-renewal and multipotency, serving as progenitors of cancer cells. The characteristics by which CSCs can be distinguished to other cancer cells are the following [53]:

1. Promotion of tumorigenesis when they are transplanted in immunosuppressed mice.
2. Expression of specific cell surface markers (such as CD44, CD133, ALDH1, CD24) and formation of tumor spheres.
3. Tumors arising from CSCs have a heterogeneous cells population composed by tumorigenic and non-tumorigenic cells.
4. Capacity of self-renewal in seriated transplants over several generations.

The presence of this subpopulation has been identified in several tumors, including HNSCC where its ability to maintain tumor population, metastasize and to be resistant to radiochemotherapy has been shown [53-55].

The origin of CSCs has not been clearly defined; in HNSCC, it has been proposed that a chronic inflammation caused by permanent tobacco, alcohol use, mechanic irritation or viral infection, in association with genetic predisposition, lead to the accumulation of various genetic alterations and finally to the manifestation of a malignant phenotype [53].

In addition, during tumor progression, some CSCs, through an EMT process, can acquire the ability to infiltrate and metastasize. On the other hand, EMT is involved in the acquisition of cancer stem cells properties; at the molecular level, the transcription factor Twist induces downregulation of E-cadherin while promoting expression of Bim1, which has an essential role in self-renewal of CSCs. In agreement with these data, high expression of Bim1 and Twist are associated with a poor prognosis in HNSCC [53].

In HNSCC patients, high percentage of CD44 positive cells was associated with higher rate of treatment failure in general, while cells expressing CD44, CD24, Oct4 and integrin β1 were associated with poor outcome after radiotherapy [56, 57]. From a clinical point of view, these evidences suggest that the patients can be cured if CSCs are completely eliminated.

3. Potential molecular markers for local recurrence and radioresistance

One of the current major research questions in the management of HNSCC disease addresses the prediction and treatment of local recurrence. As described before, mortality of patients with HNSCC is primarily driven by tumor cell radioresistance leading to local recurrence. Due to the heterogeneous nature of tumors, the identification of markers with prognostic or predictive value to be used as a complement to conventional diagnostic methods is a complex challenge. Indeed, although advance in expression technologies, current studies have provided ambiguous results.

Among the prognostic markers proposed in HNSCC, as described in the previous paragraph, the presence of mutation in *TP53* gene predicts the development of locoregional recurrence by increasing the radioresistance in tumor cells (Table 1).

Additional molecular markers predicting high local recurrence development and response to radiotherapy are summarized in Table 1.

Gene	Function	References
TP53	A tumor-suppressor regulating cell cycle progression, apoptosis and cell survival.	[2, 42, 44, 46, 58]
HIF-1α	A transcription factor induced under hypoxic condition and promoting EMT, angiogenesis, cell migration and metastasis.	[16]
PTEN	A tumor suppressor gene regulating signaling pathways controlling cell proliferation and apoptosis.	[59-62]
Fibronectin	It is a glycoprotein of the extracellular matrix, which plays a major role in cell adhesion, growth, migration, and differentiation.	[36]
EGFR	Transmembrane TK acting as a central transducer in multiple pathways that mediate cell cycle progression, angiogenesis, inhibition of apoptosis, tumor invasion and metastasis.	[14, 20]
VEGFs	Ligands of transmembrane TK promoting cell proliferation, migration and survival of endothelial cells during tumor growth.	[13, 14, 20, 51]
Cox2	Catalytic enzyme decreasing apoptosis, increasing inflammation and important for tumor progression.	[63]

Gene	Function	References
p-AKT (Ser473)	It is a serine/threonine-specific protein kinase that plays a key role in multiple cellular processes such as glucose metabolism, apoptosis, cell proliferation, transcription and cell migration.	[64]
Cyclin B1	It is a regulatory protein involved in mitosis. It begins to increase during G2, peaks in mitosis, and is rapidly degraded before the cell cycle is completed. By the interaction with cdk1, cyclin B1 promotes cell progression.	[65, 66]
E-cadherin/ Vimentin	They are protein markers of EMT; E-cadherin is a marker of epithelial cells, while vimentin is a marker of mesenchymal cells.	[34, 35]
Yap/BCL-2/ c-met/VEGF/ Clauding	They are genes involved in cell proliferation, migration, inhibition of apoptosis and angiogenesis.	[67]
Rac1	It is a member of Rac family of Rho GTPase involved in intracellular adherens junction, epithelial differentiation and regulation of motility.	[68, 69]
Pim-1	It is an oncogene with serine/threonine kinase activity mainly involved in cell cycle progression, apoptosis and transcriptional activation.	[32]
CD10	Cell surface antigen associated with CSCs.	[70]
FOXM1	It is a gene involved in cell cycle regulation, which is associated with radioresistance only in quiescent cells.	[71]
15–gene hypoxia classifier composed by ADM, ALDOA, ANKRD37, BNIP3, BNIP3L, C3orf28, EGLN3, KCTD11, LOX, NDRG1, P4HA1, P4HA2, PDK1, PFKFB3, SLC2A1	These genes are able to classify more or less hypoxic tumors. Tumors classified as high hypoxic and treated with radiotherapy show a poor outcome respect to low hypoxic ones. Accordingly, more hypoxic tumors have a better response to radiosensitiser nimorazole respect to those classified as low hypoxic.	[29]
Gene expression model of intrinsic tumor radiosensitivity based on the expression of 10 genes composed by Androgen Receptor (AR), c.Jun, STAT1, PKC, RelA, c-Abl, SUMO-1, CDK1 (p34), HDAC1, IRF1	The authors developed a radiosensitive predictive model using 10 genes comprised in central pathways involved in radioresistance. This linear regression algorithm generates a radiosensitive index RSI having a prognostic value in HNSCC datasets.	[72]

Table 1. Biomarkers predicting local recurrence and radioresistance in head and neck cancers.

3.1. MicroRNAs as new potential biomarkers predicting radiotherapy response

A class of small non-coding RNAs termed microRNAs (miRNAs) has recently been indicated as biomarker of some type of cancers [73]. miRNAs are endogenous, small, non-coding RNAs of 17-25 nucleotides that are thought to regulate approximately 30% of human genes at posttranscriptional level, primarily through their partial complementarity with the coding region or 3′ untranslated region (UTR) of target mRNAs. This leads to translational repression and/or degradation of target mRNA, therefore regulating gene expression [74]. They are involved in essential biological activities such as cellular differentiation, proliferation, development, apoptosis and cell cycle regulation. The roles of miRNAs in cancer have been extensively investigated in the past few years. The relevance of miRNAs in cancer was suggested by the observed changes in expression patterns and recurrent amplification as well as deletion of miRNA genes in cancer [75]. It has been shown that there are two types of cancer-related miRNAs: oncogenic or tumor suppressor miRNAs [74].

Several investigators have empathized the role of miRs as biomarkers for HNSCC [42] and the usefulness of miRs as prognostic factors has only begun to be explored. Moreover, miRNA expression may predict the efficacy of therapies, including radiotherapy [76]. Data from the study of miR-205 and let-7d expression showed their association with locoregional occurrence and shorter survival [77]. In addition, high expression of miR-205 can be used to detect positive lymph nodes, suggesting that this miR can be considered as a marker for metastatic HNSCC [78]. A similar study has shown that lower expression levels of miR-451 in HNSCC tumors are associated with recurrence [79]. Another recent work reported that downregulated miR-125b expression was associated with proliferation and radioresistance mechanisms, probably through ICAM2 signaling [80]. In addition, miR-17-5p expression has been shown to be induced in irradiated oral cancer cells and it downregulates p21 protein expression, contributing to radioresistance [81].

Furthermore, we also identified microRNAs signatures (miR-17-3p, miR-18b-5p, miR-324-5p, miR-19a-3p, miR-200a-3p, miR-331-3p, miR-21-3p, miR-21-5p, miR-205-5p, miR-151a-3p, miR-96-5p and miR-429) that are able to predict the risk of local recurrence and poor outcome in HNSCC tumors, and that are more powerful as biomarkers when compared to traditional prognostic indicators [42]. Finally, some evidences support the possibility to use miRNA detected in plasma as radio-responsive biomarkers for different types of cancer, including HNSCC. Accordingly, in HNSCC patients, the authors have detected changes in the abundance of circulating miRNAs (miR-425-5p and miR-93-5p) during radiochemotherapy. In addition, the researchers have demonstrated that the altered plasma miRNA changes after the therapy are the results of miRNAs release from damaged tumor cells [82].

4. Molecular strategies and future application in the treatment of HNSCC

Conventional HNSCC treatment consists of surgical resection followed by ionizing radiation or chemoradiation. In case of local advance/inoperable HNSCC, the typical treatment is concomitant platinum-based chemoradiotherapy. These standard therapies have some limitations; the surgery can result in disfigurement and functional impairment, while the radiochemotherapy, although it is an organ-preserving treatment, can cause several side effects including mucositis, oral candidiasis, loss of taste, xerostomia and osteoradionecrosis [83, 84]. In addition, overall five-year survival rate is lower than 50% in HNSCC patients. Therefore, resistance to chemoradiotherapy often occurs and is associated with recurrences and poor outcomes; this represents a major clinical problem for HNSCC patients [14].

The understanding of the molecular perturbations in the cells of carcinomas recurring after irradiation could help to identify more specific target proteins and design novel therapeutic agents that will help improving therapy outcome in patients with HNSCC recurrences.

Tumor cells repopulation is a common effect observed in radiotherapy failure. A method to decrease this phenomenon, called Accelerated Radiotherapy (AR), is the reduction of overall radiation treatment time maintaining the total dose constant [14]. This therapeutic approach has produced excellent results in patients with advanced HNSCC [85]. In addition, several studies have shown that patients overexpressing EGFR protein, result to be more sensitive and consequently to have a better response to AR [14].

Besides the modification of radiotherapy modalities, there are several therapeutic strategies, such as, for example, immunotherapy, that can be combined with radiation, and are subjected to clinical development [86] (Table 2). Currently, two of the main intriguing targets for new targeted therapy are EGFR and VEGFR [86]. Both targeted therapies can be subdivided in monoclonal antibodies and tyrosine kinase inhibitors.

4.1. EGFR targeted therapy

The role of EGFR signaling in radioresistance was widely discussed in the paragraph 2.2. Many evidences suggest that the use of EGFR inhibitors in combination with radiotherapy improves the outcomes of HNSCC patients respect to those treated with radiotherapy alone [14].

4.1.1. EGFR monoclonal antibodies

One of the main antibodies targeting EGFR is called cetuximab. Other anti-EGFR antibodies under active investigations in combination with chemoradiotherapy in HNSCC are panitumumab, zalutumumab and nimotuzumab (Table 2).

Cetuximab: It is a chimeric IgG1 mAb, which by the recognition of determinants expressed on the extracellular domain of EGFR, antagonize normal receptor interaction, preventing the activation of the downstream signaling pathways [17]. Based on the results obtained from the clinical trials, since 2006 it has been approved by the Food and Drug Administration (FDA) in association with radiotherapy [14, 86]. However, a meta-analysis studying 15 trials and focusing on the comparison of the two currently combined modality therapies show that chemoradiotherapy respect to radiotherapy plus cetuximab is associated with a better overall survival and locoregional recurrence in advanced HNSCC [87]. In addition, some HNSCC patients develop a resistance to anti-EGFR therapy mainly due to k-Ras deregulation in absence of its mutation [14, 17, 88] and the presence of the variant EGFRvIII in tumor cells [17].

In this last case, the deletion presents in this variant cause a reduction in the binding affinity of monoclonal antibodies raised with wild type EGFR [17].

Panitumumab: Preclinical evidences show that it increases radiosensitivity by the radiation-induced DNA damage and preventing the translocation of EGFR in the nucleus. Currently, therapy combining radiation in combination with panitumumab is undergoing phase III clinical trials [86]. In addition, a phase III trial performed in advanced HNSCC patients to compare 5-FU and cisplatin treatment in presence and not of panitumumab have not shown an important improvement of the clinical outcome [89].

Zalutumumab: Several studies on phase I/II trial were performed using this drug at different doses in combination to radiation and/or chemotherapy; the results are encouraging and a phase III is ongoing [86].

Nimotuzumab: Preclinical studies show that it has antiproliferative, antiangiogenic and proapoptotic effects and it is well tolerated in HNSCC patients treated with radiation [86]. However, it has been demonstrated that cetuximab is more effective in comparison to nimotuzumab in enhancing radiosensitivity in high-EGFR expressing cells [90].

In conclusion, antibody anti-EGFR in combination with radiation therapy was well tolerated in HNSCC patients; currently, the best-studied mAb are cetuximab and panitumumab. Both improve radiosensitivity and overall survival in advanced HNSCC treated with radiation. However, the addition of cetuximab to conventional chemoradiotherapy has not shown a significant improvement in clinical outcome and the results obtained from the treatment of a large number of patients in multi-centered trials has shown that the treatment is effective in about 20% of cases [17].

To date, the use of cetuximab in combination with radiation represents a standard clinical approach, particularly in HNSCC patients who cannot tolerate chemotherapy [86].

4.1.2. EGFR tyrosine kinase inhibitors

Another group of agents targeting EGFR are small molecule tyrosine kinase inhibitors (TKIs). They act preventing EGFR autophosphorylation and consequently its activation by the occupation of the EGFR intracellular ATP-binding domain [17]. The two best studied TKIs are gefitinib (Iressa) and erlotinib (Tarceva). Others are called lapatinib and afanitib (Table 2).

Gefitinib: Preclinical studies show that gefitinib treatment on HNSCC cells can inhibit cell proliferation, decrease cell survival and enhance tumor cell radiosensitivity [91]. In addition, encouraging results were obtained in the clinical studies when gefitinib was combined with VEGFR inhibitors or other targets, suggesting the possibility to use it as possible neoadjuvant agent. Besides that, clinical trials combining gefitinib with chemoradiotherapy have not yet demonstrated a significant improvement respect to conventional therapy [86].

Erlotinib: Encouraging results were obtained from preclinical studies showing that the combination of erlotinib with radiation and/or VEGFR inhibitors improve treatment efficacy by the inhibition of tumor growth, proliferation and vessel density [92, 93]. However, to date, there is no convincing clinical evidence that the addition of erlotinib to conventional therapy is universally beneficial [86]

Lapatinib and Afatinib: They are orally active EGFR and HER2 inhibitors, which seem to be well tolerated from HNSCC patients. Interestingly, in p16-negative HNSCC patients, a large difference in clinical outcome was observed in patients treated with lapatinib versus placebo. Phase III trials are ongoing in HNSCC for both molecules [86].

4.2. VEGF targeted therapy

As explained in the paragraph 2.5, VEGF is one of the most important regulators of angiogenesis; its upregulation is a common event in HNSCC and it is associated with radioresistance and poor prognosis.

4.2.1. VEGF monoclonal antibodies

Bevacizumab (Avastin) (Table 2) is the main recombinant anti-VEGFA monoclonal antibody under active investigation for HNSCC therapy. Preclinical evidences show that bevacizumab is able to act as radiation sensitizer in HNSCC cells, to reduce angiogenesis and tumor growth [86]. Phase I/II clinical trials performed using bevacizumab in combination with conventional chemoradiotherapy in HNSCC have shown that although this combined modality therapy is possible, to date there is no strong evidence that the addition of bevacizumab to chemoradiotherapy causes an improvement of the overall survival in HNSCC patients [13]. Future investigations are necessary to define the effectiveness of this molecule in the treatment of HNSCC.

4.2.2. VEGFR tyrosine kinase inhibitors

To date, the known VEGF tyrosine kinase inhibitors are: vandetanib (ZD6474), sunitinib, sorafenib and linifanib (ABT-869) (Table 2).

Vandetanib: It is an orally multi-kinase inhibitor targeting EGFR, VEGFR-2 and RET tyrosine kinases. Preclinical evidences show that the administration of vandetanib enhances the antitumor effects of radiation therapy by inhibition of both EGFR and VEGFR signaling in HNSCC human tumor xenografts; in particular, the authors demonstrate that radiation plus vandetanib treatment is effective in both overexpressing EGFR tumor cells and EGFR- null cells [94]. In addition, vandetanib restores HNSCC cells sensitivity to cisplatin and radiation *in vivo* and *in vitro* by promoting an increase of apoptosis and a decrease of microvessel density [95]. A randomized phase II clinical trial using a combination of cisplatin and radiation with or without vandetanib in advanced HNSCC is under consideration [13].

Sunitinib: It is an orally multi-kinase inhibitor targeting VEGFR, PDGFR and c-Kit tyrosine kinases. Preclinical and clinical studies show that sunitinib has low activity as monotherapy, but in combination with cetuximab and radiation, it causes a strong tumor inhibition effect by a complete abolition of tumor growth. Specifically, the combination of cetuximab and sunitinib causes a decrease of cell proliferation and enhances cell differentiation, while a decrease in tumor vessels number was observed when the radiation treatment was added [96]. These results encourage future clinical investigations regarding the sunitinib and chemoradiotherapy treatment combination.

Sorafenib: It is an oral inhibitor of serine/threonine protein kinase b-Raf, C-Raf, VEGFR and PDGFR. Preclinical evidences show that sorafenib in combination with chemoradiation is able to enhance a more effective antitumor effect by the inhibition of cell growth, clone formation, cell migration and invasion compared to chemoradiation or radiation alone. This therapy combination is also able to inhibit tumor angiogenesis [97]. In addition, sunitinib can increase the antiproliferative effect of chemoradiotherapy by inhibiting the Raf/MEK/ERK signaling pathway and consequently downregulating the expression of the DNA repair proteins ERCC-1 and XRCC-1 [13]. Although these results suggest that sorafenib could enhance the effectiveness of chemoradiotherapy, ongoing phase I/II clinical trials will determine the real efficacy of sorafenib in HNSCC patients.

Linifanib: It is a novel ATP-competitive tyrosine kinase inhibitor of the VEGF and PDGF receptor family members. Preliminary data on HNSCC cells show that linifanib can act as radiation sensitizer since its combination with radiation is more effective compared to radiation or chemoradiation alone [13].

4.3. Other targeted therapies

As explained in the paragraph 2 relative to molecular mechanisms of radioresistance, there are many actors playing a key role in the failure of radiotherapy in HNSCC. As a consequence, targeted therapies against other molecules besides EGFR and VEGF family proteins were developed and their characterization is still ongoing. Among them, there are Src-family kinase inhibitors such as dosatinib; proteasome inhibitors as bortezomib, cyclooxygenase(Cox)-2 inhibitor (colecoxib); PI3K/Akt/mTOR inhibitors as wortmannin, perifostine and temsirolimus; and therapies targeting c-Met signaling pathway [14, 86] (Table 2).

Briefly, Src-kinase inhibitor dasatinib promotes radiosensitization by decreasing EGFR phosphorylation, its translocation in the nucleus and consequently, its association with DNA–protein kinases, blocking DNA repair pathways [98, 99]. Evidences on proteasome inhibitor bortezomib show its capability to act as radiosensitizer; specifically, it promotes the upregulation of PTEN activity and downregulation of p-Akt, leading to an increase of apoptosis of tumor cells [100-102]. Cox inhibitor colecoxib leads to a decrease of VEGFR expression and angiogenesis [103]. Next, mTOR inhibitors cause a reduction of angiogenesis and an induction of cell death by autophagy [86, 104]. Finally, given the important role discussed in the paragraph 2 on the significance of CSCs subpopulation in radioresistance, an emerging concept is the combined use of standard chemoradiotherapy with cancer stem cells targeted therapy. Preclinical study on CD44 expressing HNSCC cells combine radiation with anti-CD44 antibodies; the results show an increase in local tumor control in patients treated with radiation plus anti-CD44 antibodies compared to those treated with radiation alone in vivo [105].

Anticancer Agent	Type of agent	Target of Agent	Phase of development in HNSCC
Cetuximab	mAb IgG1	EGFR	Approved by FDA, phase III/IV
Panitumumab	mAb IgG2	EGFR	Phase III
Zalutumumab	mAb IgG1	EGFR	Phase III
Nimotuzumab	mAb	EGFR	Phase III
Gefitinib	TKI	EGFR	Phase I/II
Erlotinib	TKI	EGFR	Phase I/II
Afatinib	TKI	EGFR/HER2	Phase III
Lapatinib	TKI	EGFR/HER2	Phase III
Bevacizumab	mAb	VEGFA	Phase III
Vandetanib	TKI	VEGFR/EGFR	Phase I
Sunitinib	TKI	VEGFR/PDGFR/kit	Phase I
Sorafenib	TKI	VEGFR/PDGFR/Raf	Phase I
MM-121	mAb IgG2	HER-2	Preclinical phase
Pertuzumab	mAb IgG1	HER-3	Preclinical phase
AV-203	mAb IgG1	HER-3	Phase I
RO5479599	mAb	HER-3	Preclinical phase
Motesanib	TKI	VEGFR/PDGFR/kit	Preclinical phase
Dasatinib	TKI	Src family kinase	Phase I/II
Bortezomib	Proteasome inhibitor	26S proteasome	Phase I
Celecoxib	Nonsteroidal anti-inflammatory inhibitor	Cox-2	Phase I
Everolimus	Inhibitor derived from rapamycin	mTor	Phase I
Temsirolimus	Inhibitor derived from rapamycin	mTor	Phase I
Onartuzumab	mAb	c-Met	Preclinical phase
Cixutumumab	mAB IgG1	IGFR	Phase 0/II
Ficlatuzumab	mAb IgG1	HGF	Phase I
AMG 102	mAb IgG2	HGF	Preclinical phase
Fresolimumab	mAb IgG4	TGF-β	Preclinical phase

Table 2. List of molecular targeted therapies combined with radiotherapy under consideration for treatment of HNSCC patients (clinicaltrials.gov) [13, 86, 106].

4.4. Therapy by reactivation or elimination of mutant p53 protein

The vast majority of HNSCC show mutations in *TP53* gene; several evidences have shown that mutant p53 protein loses its function as tumor suppressor and acquires new oncogenic functions by which it promotes resistance to cisplatin and radiation treatment. The transfection of wild-type *TP53* into cell lines induces growth arrest and reduces tumorigenicity in nude mice. This suggested that restoring p53 function in HNSCC could inhibit cell growth [107]. HNSCC has been one of the first tumor localities to benefit from gene transfer therapy. Several strategies have been developed to restore p53 function in HNSCC [14, 108].

Gene therapy: The most used vector for p53 gene therapy in HNSCC is the adenovirus, for its high affinity with the cells of the upper aerodigestive tract. A series of modified p53 adenoviruses (Ad-p53) are able to induce apoptosis and sensitize HNSCC cells to radiotherapy [109, 110]. Therefore, a phase I/II clinical trial based on the injection of Ad-p53 in HNSCC patients was performed and has shown that Ad-p53 is a promising therapeutic strategy [111, 112]. A phase III study based on the comparison of Ad-p53 to methotrexate treatment in advanced HNSCC show that overall, there is no significant difference in clinical outcome between these two subgroups of treated HNSCC, but, interestingly, Ad-p53 treatment was associated with a significant increase of survival in specific subgroup of HNSCC patients, having *TP53* wild type but inactivated by the upregulation of p53 inhibitors Mdm-2 or Mdm-4 [113]. This evidence suggests the possibility to select HNSCC patients who are most likely to benefit from Ad-p53 therapy. Another phase III clinical trial based on the use of recombinant Ad-p53 (gendicine) injection in combination with radiation shows encouraging results [114].

Virus targeting p53 deficient cells: This therapeutic strategy is based on the elimination of mutant p53. The efficient replication of adenovirus requires the neutralization of p53 function through E1B viral protein. ONYX-015 is an engineered adenovirus that does not express E1B protein and consequently is able to induce viral replication and cell death only in tumor cells carrying *TP53* mutations. Phase I/II clinical trials performed in HNSCC patients have shown that intravenous administration of ONYX-15 is feasible and while the treatment with ONYX-15 alone gave only marginal effects, its combination with cisplatin and 5-fluorouracil had a more profound impact on the response of patients [115]. Other clinical trials will be necessary to evaluate its real effectiveness in HNSCC treatment.

Molecules reactivating mutant p53: They are small molecules able to alter the conformation of mutant p53 to wild type, leading to the restoration of its tumor suppression function. Among them, glycerol treatment is able to reactivate p53 wild-type functions in HNSCC cell lines carrying mutant p53 by its ability to refold proteins [116]. Due to its toxicity, glycerol use is not so feasible in HNSCC patients. As a consequence, a series of other similar molecules was developed. Among them, PRIMA and CP-31389 were tested in HNSCC cell lines carrying mutant p53 and have demonstrated to inhibit proliferation and promote apoptosis by the induction of p53-related genes expression, including p21, Bax, Puma and Noxa [117]. Currently, there are no clinical data testing real effectiveness of these molecules in the treatment of HNSCC patients.

Molecules disrupting p53 inhibitors: In tumor cells, the function of p53 protein can be compromised not only by the presence of mutation on its gene, but also by upregulation of its inhibitors. The main p53 natural inhibitor is MDM2, which functions binding p53 protein and promoting its degradation. Nutlins and their derivate RITA are a class of small molecules able to prevent the binding MDM2-p53, restoring p53 tumor suppressor function. Therefore, Nutlins and RITA treatment leads to an increase of nuclear p53 levels, inhibition of proliferation, increase of cell death and antitumor efficacy of cisplatin [108]. Therapy treatment based on these molecules is more effective in tumor cells carrying p53 wild-type compared with mutant p53-carrying cells.

In addition, in a subset of HPV-related HNSCC, the activity of p53 can be also inhibited by the exogenous viral oncoprotein E6. Specifically, it acts by interacting with E6AP protein to degrade p53 via proteasome pathway and with p300 to prevent p53 acetylation. Treatment of HNSCC cell lines with the small molecule CH1iB, disrupting the binding of E6 HPV16 protein and p300, promotes an increase of the p53 acetylation levels and therefore an increase of p53 transcriptional activity. Additionally, Ch1iB shows an anticancer effect also due to its capability to reduce cancer stem cells population and by sensitizing tumor cells to cisplatin treatment in HPV positive cells [14, 108].

4.5. microRNAs as therapeutic agents

The role of microRNAs as predictors and modifiers of chemoradiotherapy in several kinds of human cancers, including HNSCC, has been shown [118]. For instance, miR-125b transfection on oral cancer cell lines enhances radiosensitivity to X-ray irradiation [80]. In addition, changes in the abundance of circulating miRNAs during radiochemotherapy has been detected and has been shown to reflect the therapy response of primary HNSCC cells after an in vitro treatment [82]. Finally, in our laboratory, we have demonstrated that the expression of signatures of *TP53* mutation-associated miRNAs, composed of 12 and 4 miRNAs, predicts, respectively, the risk of local recurrence insurgence and poor outcome, independently from other relevant prognostic indicators [42]. These evidences suggest the possibility of monitoring changes in miRNAs expression before to and during treatment in order to estimate the effectiveness of certain therapies. At the same time, another possibility for future application of miRNAs in therapy is the modulation of deregulated miRNAs concentration by molecules that replace downregulated miRNAs or using antagonists that binds overexpressed miRNAs [119]. Evidence supporting this possibility has been shown for the treatment of HCV infection; this phase II clinical study is based on the treatment of HCV infected patients with Miravirsen by which miR-122 is sequestered [120]. Miravirsen is the first miR-targeted drug to receive Investigation New Drug (IND) acceptance from FDA [121]. To date, there is only one clinical trial available in cancer patients; in particular, the treatment of liver cancer with MRX34, which is a molecule mimicking miR-34, is ongoing, in order to evaluate its maximum tolerated dose and its pharmacokinetics in patients [119].

4.6. TRAIL and Smac mimetics molecules

Recently, two classes of novel therapeutic agents targeting specific molecules involved in apoptosis pathway have emerged. The first one is the tumor necrosis factor-related apoptosis-inducing ligand (TRAIL). It is able to induce cell death by binding to its corresponding cell surface receptor TRAIL-R1/R2 and activating the apoptotic pathways [122-124]. A second class of targeted anticancer agents is composed by Smac mimetics (SMs). They mimic the function of endogenous proapoptotic mitochondrial protein Smac/Diablo [125]. In response to a death stimulus, it is released in the cytoplasm and inhibits the antiapoptotic activity of IAP proteins

[126]. Both TRAIL and SMs have been tested in several cancer models [123, 125, 127]. A study testing the sensitivity to TRAIL and SMs treatment on HNSCC cell lines show that both molecules are highly effective in killing tumor cells. In addition, caspase 8 and TNF-α expression was identified as biomarker for predicting, respectively, TRAIL and SMs sensitivity [128]. These preliminary results encourage future investigations on the possibility to use them as targeted HNSCC treatment.

4.7. Therapeutic activity of molecules derived from plants

Antineoplastic effects of molecules derived from plant extracts have recently gained increasing attention as an additive to traditional therapies of cancer, including HNSCC.

One of the most studied molecules derived from plants for HNSCC treatment is curcumin (diferuloylmethane). It is a polyphenol derived from the *Curcuma longa* plant, commonly known as turmeric. Curcumin, which has been used extensively in Ayurvedic medicine for centuries, is a pleiotropic molecule able to interact with multiple molecular targets and signal transduction pathways, and has a variety of therapeutic properties, including antioxidant, analgesic, anti-inflammatory and antiseptic activity [15]. More recently, curcumin has been found to possess anti-cancer activities, acting on several biological pathways involved in mutagenesis, oncogene expression, cell cycle regulation, apoptosis, tumorigenesis and metastasis [15]. For instance, it is able to inhibit the transcription factor NF-kB and downstream gene products (including c-myc, bcl-2, COX-2, NOS, cyclin D1, TNF-alpha, interleukins and MMP-9). Additionally, curcumin affects a variety of growth factor receptors and cell adhesion molecules involved in tumor growth, angiogenesis and metastasis [15]. As a natural product, curcumin is no toxic. It is a potent antitumor agent also in HNSCC and can be used to overcome chemoradiotherapy resistance. Indeed, the treatment of HNSCC cell lines with a molecule derived from curcumin (H-4073) inhibits cell proliferation, angiogenesis and significantly sensitizes the cells to cisplatin treatment. H-4073 mediated its antitumor effects by inhibiting JAK/STAT3, FAK, Akt and VEGF signaling pathways that play important role in cell proliferation, migration, survival and angiogenesis [129]. Another study shows that curcumin sensitizes to radiation HPV-negative HNSCC cells with high levels of Thioredoxin reductase (TrxRs). Indeed, in this work it has been demonstrated that the efficacy of curcumin in sensitizing tumor cells to radiation depends on its ability to inhibit TrxRd1. TrxRs are a family of NADPH-dependent flavoproteins, which are involved in several redox-regulated cellular functions as transcription, DNA repair, proliferation, angiogenesis and apoptosis. Specifically, high levels of TrxRd1 isoform were found in HNSCC and were associated with poor outcome [130]. Finally, data from a very recent study shows that curcumin is more effective, in terms of inhibition of cancer growth, when combined with another non-flavonoid polyphenol called Resveratrol [131].

Another intriguing natural anticancer Chinese medicine is Gamboge. It acts as anti-inflammatory agent, detoxifying and apoptotic inducer in different type of cancer cells. Interestingly, the Gamboge derivate Compound 2 (C2) is able to inhibit growth also in HNSCC stem cells. Indeed, it can inhibit formation of tumor spheres and repress the expression of multiples genes related to cancer stem cell phenotype by blocking the activation of EGFR pathways [132]. Since one of the main causes of failure in HNSCC treatment is the enrichment of CSCs population, which are resistant to current therapy, the future use of this molecule in combination with chemoradiotherapy could prevent the selective enrichment of CSCs after HNSCC conventional treatment.

5. Conclusions

Radioresistance strongly affects the clinical outcome of HNSCC patients. The key mechanisms by which radioresistance occur have been associated with deregulation of several molecular signaling pathways such as EGFR, VEGFR and p53. Recently, it has been shown that the enrichment of a small population of tumor cells, named cancer stem cells, also plays an important role in the failure of conventional HNSCC treatment. In addition, current treatments are associated with high toxicity and side effects. The basis of treatment decisions are mainly based on TNM staging, but patients with the same staging have different response to therapy. Several molecular targeted therapies are actively under investigation in order to improve the effectiveness of current therapy. Only a few of these strategies have been tested in clinical trials and to date cetuximab is the unique targeted therapy approved from FDA. However, this treatment showed efficacy in about 20% of HNSCC patients. In addition, due to the heterogeneous nature of these tumors, the study of molecular prognostic and predictive factors has been motivated by the necessity to predict radiosensitivity of patients and to define more homogenous groups of patients for treatment selection. Indeed, personalized treatment plans based on biomarkers could improve overall survival and reduce morbidity. Although several evidences have shown that many molecules, as proteins and microRNAs, can potentially predict response to therapy and clinical outcome, to date, the HNSCC treatment decision is uniquely based on TNM staging and HPV infection. One of the reasons of the difficulties to find efficacious biomarkers is the disagreement between these studies; this mainly relies on the variety of tumor sites, sensitivity of the techniques used, quality of the specimens studied and the arbitrary cut-off values set.

Author details

Federica Ganci[1], Andrea Sacconi[1], Valentina Manciocco[1], Giuseppe Spriano[1], Giulia Fontemaggi[1], Paolo Carlini[2] and Giovanni Blandino[1*]

*Address all correspondence to: blandino@ifo.it

1 Translational Oncogenomics Unit, National Cancer Institute "Regina Elena", Rome, Italy

2 Medical Oncology A, National Cancer Institute "Regina Elena", Rome, Italy

References

[1] Mitra S, Banerjee S, Misra C, Singh RK, Roy A, Sengupta A, et al. Interplay between human papilloma virus infection and p53 gene alterations in head and neck squamous cell carcinoma of an Indian patient population. Journal of clinical pathology. 2007;60(9):1040-7. Epub 2006/11/03.

[2] Leemans CR, Braakhuis BJ, Brakenhoff RH. The molecular biology of head and neck cancer. Nature reviews cancer. 2011;11(1):9-22. Epub 2010/12/17.

[3] Ragin CC, Modugno F, Gollin SM. The epidemiology and risk factors of head and neck cancer: a focus on human papillomavirus. Journal of dental research. 2007;86(2): 104-14. Epub 2007/01/26.

[4] Talamini R, Bosetti C, La Vecchia C, Dal Maso L, Levi F, Bidoli E, et al. Combined effect of tobacco and alcohol on laryngeal cancer risk: a case-control study. Cancer causes & control : CCC. 2002;13(10):957-64. Epub 2003/02/18.

[5] Werbrouck J, De Ruyck K, Duprez F, Van Eijkeren M, Rietzschel E, Bekaert S, et al. Single-nucleotide polymorphisms in DNA double-strand break repair genes: association with head and neck cancer and interaction with tobacco use and alcohol consumption. Mutation research. 2008;656(1-2):74-81. Epub 2008/09/05.

[6] Chung CH, Gillison ML. Human papillomavirus in head and neck cancer: its role in pathogenesis and clinical implications. Clinical cancer research : an official journal of the American Association for Cancer Research. 2009;15(22):6758-62. Epub 2009/10/29.

[7] D'Souza G, Kreimer AR, Viscidi R, Pawlita M, Fakhry C, Koch WM, et al. Case-control study of human papillomavirus and oropharyngeal cancer. The New England journal of medicine. 2007;356(19):1944-56. Epub 2007/05/15.

[8] Choi P, Chen C. Genetic expression profiles and biologic pathway alterations in head and neck squamous cell carcinoma. Cancer. 2005;104(6):1113-28. Epub 2005/08/11.

[9] Sahu N, Grandis JR. New advances in molecular approaches to head and neck squamous cell carcinoma. Anti-cancer drugs. 2011;22(7):656-64. Epub 2010/12/24.

[10] Lambrecht M, Dirix P, Van den Bogaert W, Nuyts S. Incidence of isolated regional recurrence after definitive chemoradiotherapy for head and neck squamous cell carcinoma. Radiotherapy and oncology : journal of the European Society for Therapeutic Radiology and Oncology. 2009;93(3):498-502. Epub 2009/09/22.

[11] Ha PK, Califano JA. The molecular biology of mucosal field cancerization of the head and neck. Critical reviews in oral biology and medicine : an official publication of the American Association of Oral Biologists. 2003;14(5):363-9. Epub 2003/10/08.

[12] Braakhuis BJ, Tabor MP, Kummer JA, Leemans CR, Brakenhoff RH. A genetic explanation of Slaughter's concept of field cancerization: evidence and clinical implications. Cancer research. 2003;63(8):1727-30. Epub 2003/04/19.

[13] Hsu HW, Wall NR, Hsueh CT, Kim S, Ferris RL, Chen CS, et al. Combination antiangiogenic therapy and radiation in head and neck cancers. Oral oncology. 2014;50(1): 19-26. Epub 2013/11/26.

[14] Perri F, Pacelli R, Della Vittoria Scarpati G, Cella L, Giuliano M, Caponigro F, et al. Radioresistance in head and neck squamous cell carcinoma: biological bases and therapeutic implications. Head & neck. 2014. Epub 2014/07/06.

[15] Wilken R, Veena MS, Wang MB, Srivatsan ES. Curcumin: a review of anti-cancer properties and therapeutic activity in head and neck squamous cell carcinoma. Molecular cancer. 2011;10:12. Epub 2011/02/09.

[16] Meijer TW, Kaanders JH, Span PN, Bussink J. Targeting hypoxia, HIF-1, and tumor glucose metabolism to improve radiotherapy efficacy. Clinical cancer research : an official journal of the American Association for Cancer Research. 2012;18(20):5585-94. Epub 2012/10/17.

[17] Sharafinski ME, Ferris RL, Ferrone S, Grandis JR. Epidermal growth factor receptor targeted therapy of squamous cell carcinoma of the head and neck. Head & neck. 2010;32(10):1412-21. Epub 2010/09/18.

[18] Kizaka-Kondoh S, Inoue M, Harada H, Hiraoka M. Tumor hypoxia: a target for selective cancer therapy. Cancer science. 2003;94(12):1021-8. Epub 2003/12/10.

[19] Nordsmark M, Bentzen SM, Rudat V, Brizel D, Lartigau E, Stadler P, et al. Prognostic value of tumor oxygenation in 397 head and neck tumors after primary radiation therapy. An international multi-center study. Radiotherapy and oncology : journal of the European Society for Therapeutic Radiology and Oncology. 2005;77(1):18-24. Epub 2005/08/16.

[20] Nijkamp MM, Span PN, Bussink J, Kaanders JH. Interaction of EGFR with the tumour microenvironment: implications for radiation treatment. Radiotherapy and oncology : journal of the European Society for Therapeutic Radiology and Oncology. 2013;108(1):17-23. Epub 2013/06/12.

[21] Harris AL. Hypoxia--a key regulatory factor in tumour growth. Nature reviews cancer. 2002;2(1):38-47. Epub 2002/03/21.

[22] Wachsberger P, Burd R, Dicker AP. Tumor response to ionizing radiation combined with antiangiogenesis or vascular targeting agents: exploring mechanisms of interaction. Clinical cancer research : an official journal of the American Association for Cancer Research. 2003;9(6):1957-71. Epub 2003/06/11.

[23] Hoff CM. Importance of hemoglobin concentration and its modification for the outcome of head and neck cancer patients treated with radiotherapy. Acta Oncol. 2012;51(4):419-32. Epub 2012/02/09.

[24] Chapman JD. Measurement of tumor hypoxia by invasive and non-invasive procedures: a review of recent clinical studies. Radiotherapy and oncology : journal of the European Society for Therapeutic Radiology and Oncology. 1991;20 (Suppl 1):13-9. Epub 1991/01/01.

[25] Hodgkiss RJ. Use of 2-nitroimidazoles as bioreductive markers for tumour hypoxia. Anti-cancer drug design. 1998;13(6):687-702. Epub 1998/10/02.

[26] Koukourakis MI, Giatromanolaki A, Sivridis E, Simopoulos C, Turley H, Talks K, et al. Hypoxia-inducible factor (HIF1A and HIF2A), angiogenesis, and chemoradiotherapy outcome of squamous cell head-and-neck cancer. International journal of radiation oncology, biology, physics. 2002;53(5):1192-202. Epub 2002/07/20.

[27] Koukourakis MI, Giatromanolaki A, Sivridis E, Simopoulos K, Pastorek J, Wykoff CC, et al. Hypoxia-regulated carbonic anhydrase-9 (CA9) relates to poor vascularization and resistance of squamous cell head and neck cancer to chemoradiotherapy. Clinical cancer research : an official journal of the American Association for Cancer Research. 2001;7(11):3399-403. Epub 2001/11/14.

[28] Toustrup K, Sorensen BS, Lassen P, Wiuf C, Alsner J, Overgaard J. Gene expression classifier predicts for hypoxic modification of radiotherapy with nimorazole in squamous cell carcinomas of the head and neck. Radiotherapy and oncology : journal of the European Society for Therapeutic Radiology and Oncology. 2012;102(1):122-9. Epub 2011/10/15.

[29] Toustrup K, Sorensen BS, Nordsmark M, Busk M, Wiuf C, Alsner J, et al. Development of a hypoxia gene expression classifier with predictive impact for hypoxic modification of radiotherapy in head and neck cancer. Cancer research. 2011;71(17): 5923-31. Epub 2011/08/19.

[30] Winter SC, Buffa FM, Silva P, Miller C, Valentine HR, Turley H, et al. Relation of a hypoxia metagene derived from head and neck cancer to prognosis of multiple cancers. Cancer research. 2007;67(7):3441-9. Epub 2007/04/06.

[31] Lo HW, Hung MC. Nuclear EGFR signalling network in cancers: linking EGFR pathway to cell cycle progression, nitric oxide pathway and patient survival. British journal of cancer. 2006;94(2):184-8. Epub 2006/01/26.

[32] Peltola K, Hollmen M, Maula SM, Rainio E, Ristamaki R, Luukkaa M, et al. Pim-1 kinase expression predicts radiation response in squamocellular carcinoma of head and neck and is under the control of epidermal growth factor receptor. Neoplasia. 2009;11(7):629-36. Epub 2009/07/02.

[33] Scanlon CS, Van Tubergen EA, Inglehart RC, D'Silva NJ. Biomarkers of epithelial-mesenchymal transition in squamous cell carcinoma. Journal of dental research. 2013;92(2):114-21. Epub 2012/11/07.

[34] Zhao Z, Ge J, Sun Y, Tian L, Lu J, Liu M, et al. Is E-cadherin immunoexpression a prognostic factor for head and neck squamous cell carcinoma (HNSCC)? A systematic review and meta-analysis. Oral oncology. 2012;48(9):761-7. Epub 2012/03/30.

[35] Liu LK, Jiang XY, Zhou XX, Wang DM, Song XL, Jiang HB. Upregulation of vimentin and aberrant expression of E-cadherin/beta-catenin complex in oral squamous cell carcinomas: correlation with the clinicopathological features and patient outcome. Modern pathology : an official journal of the United States and Canadian Academy of Pathology, Inc. 2010;23(2):213-24. Epub 2009/11/17.

[36] Jerhammar F, Ceder R, Garvin S, Grenman R, Grafstrom RC, Roberg K. Fibronectin 1 is a potential biomarker for radioresistance in head and neck squamous cell carcinoma. Cancer biology & therapy. 2010;10(12):1244-51. Epub 2010/10/12.

[37] Olivier M, Hollstein M, Hainaut P. TP53 mutations in human cancers: origins, consequences, and clinical use. Cold Spring Harbor perspectives in biology. 2010;2(1):a001008. Epub 2010/02/26.

[38] Di Agostino S, Strano S, Emiliozzi V, Zerbini V, Mottolese M, Sacchi A, et al. Gain of function of mutant p53: the mutant p53/NF-Y protein complex reveals an aberrant transcriptional mechanism of cell cycle regulation. Cancer cell. 2006;10(3):191-202. Epub 2006/09/09.

[39] Fontemaggi G, Dell'Orso S, Trisciuoglio D, Shay T, Melucci E, Fazi F, et al. The execution of the transcriptional axis mutant p53, E2F1 and ID4 promotes tumor neo-angiogenesis. Nature structural & molecular biology. 2009;16(10):1086-93. Epub 2009/09/29.

[40] Obata A, Eura M, Sasaki J, Saya H, Chikamatsu K, Tada M, et al. Clinical significance of p53 functional loss in squamous cell carcinoma of the oropharynx. International journal of cancer/Journal international du cancer. 2000;89(2):187-93. Epub 2001/02/07.

[41] Alsner J, Sorensen SB, Overgaard J. TP53 mutation is related to poor prognosis after radiotherapy, but not surgery, in squamous cell carcinoma of the head and neck. Radiotherapy and oncology : journal of the European Society for Therapeutic Radiology and Oncology. 2001;59(2):179-85. Epub 2001/04/28.

[42] Ganci F, Sacconi A, Bossel Ben-Moshe N, Manciocco V, Sperduti I, Strigari L, et al. Expression of TP53 mutation-associated microRNAs predicts clinical outcome in head and neck squamous cell carcinoma patients. Annals of oncology : official journal of the European Society for Medical Oncology / ESMO. 2013;24(12):3082-8. Epub 2013/10/11.

[43] Gross AM, Orosco RK, Shen JP, Egloff AM, Carter H, Hofree M, et al. Multi-tiered genomic analysis of head and neck cancer ties TP53 mutation to 3p loss. Nature genetics. 2014;46(9):939-43. Epub 2014/08/05.

[44] Poeta ML, Manola J, Goldwasser MA, Forastiere A, Benoit N, Califano JA, et al. TP53 mutations and survival in squamous-cell carcinoma of the head and neck. The New England journal of medicine. 2007;357(25):2552-61. Epub 2007/12/21.

[45] Peltonen JK, Vahakangas KH, Helppi HM, Bloigu R, Paakko P, Turpeenniemi-Hujanen T. Specific TP53 mutations predict aggressive phenotype in head and neck squamous cell carcinoma: a retrospective archival study. Head & neck oncology. 2011;3:20. Epub 2011/04/26.

[46] Skinner HD, Sandulache VC, Ow TJ, Meyn RE, Yordy JS, Beadle BM, et al. TP53 disruptive mutations lead to head and neck cancer treatment failure through inhibition of radiation-induced senescence. Clinical cancer research : an official journal of the American Association for Cancer Research. 2012;18(1):290-300. Epub 2011/11/18.

[47] Lehmann BD, McCubrey JA, Jefferson HS, Paine MS, Chappell WH, Terrian DM. A dominant role for p53-dependent cellular senescence in radiosensitization of human prostate cancer cells. Cell Cycle. 2007;6(5):595-605. Epub 2007/03/14.

[48] Kleibeuker EA, Griffioen AW, Verheul HM, Slotman BJ, Thijssen VL. Combining angiogenesis inhibition and radiotherapy: a double-edged sword. Drug resistance updates : reviews and commentaries in antimicrobial and anticancer chemotherapy. 2012;15(3):173-82. Epub 2012/05/09.

[49] Ferrara N, Gerber HP, LeCouter J. The biology of VEGF and its receptors. Nature medicine. 2003;9(6):669-76. Epub 2003/06/05.

[50] Kyzas PA, Cunha IW, Ioannidis JP. Prognostic significance of vascular endothelial growth factor immunohistochemical expression in head and neck squamous cell carcinoma: a meta-analysis. Clinical cancer research : an official journal of the American Association for Cancer Research. 2005;11(4):1434-40. Epub 2005/03/05.

[51] Brieger J, Kattwinkel J, Berres M, Gosepath J, Mann WJ. Impact of vascular endothelial growth factor release on radiation resistance. Oncology reports. 2007;18(6): 1597-601. Epub 2007/11/06.

[52] Clarke MF, Fuller M. Stem cells and cancer: two faces of eve. Cell. 2006;124(6):1111-5. Epub 2006/03/28.

[53] Satpute PS, Hazarey V, Ahmed R, Yadav L. Cancer stem cells in head and neck squamous cell carcinoma: a review. Asian Pacific journal of cancer prevention : APJCP. 2013;14(10):5579-87. Epub 2013/12/03.

[54] Allegra E, Trapasso S. Cancer stem cells in head and neck cancer. OncoTargets and therapy. 2012;5:375-83. Epub 2012/11/29.

[55] Prince ME, Sivanandan R, Kaczorowski A, Wolf GT, Kaplan MJ, Dalerba P, et al. Identification of a subpopulation of cells with cancer stem cell properties in head and neck squamous cell carcinoma. Proceedings of the National Academy of Sciences of the United States of America. 2007;104(3):973-8. Epub 2007/01/11.

[56] Joshua B, Kaplan MJ, Doweck I, Pai R, Weissman IL, Prince ME, et al. Frequency of cells expressing CD44, a head and neck cancer stem cell marker: correlation with tumor aggressiveness. Head & neck. 2012;34(1):42-9. Epub 2011/02/16.

[57] Koukourakis MI, Giatromanolaki A, Tsakmaki V, Danielidis V, Sivridis E. Cancer stem cell phenotype relates to radio-chemotherapy outcome in locally advanced squamous cell head-neck cancer. British journal of cancer. 2012;106(5):846-53. Epub 2012/02/16.

[58] Thomas GR, Nadiminti H, Regalado J. Molecular predictors of clinical outcome in patients with head and neck squamous cell carcinoma. International journal of experimental pathology. 2005;86(6):347-63. Epub 2005/11/29.

[59] Mriouah J, Boura C, Pinel S, Chretien AS, Fifre A, Merlin JL, et al. Cellular response to cetuximab in PTEN-silenced head and neck squamous cell carcinoma cell line. International journal of oncology. 2010;37(6):1555-63. Epub 2010/11/03.

[60] Pai SI, Westra WH. Molecular pathology of head and neck cancer: implications for diagnosis, prognosis, and treatment. Annual review of pathology. 2009;4:49-70. Epub 2008/08/30.

[61] Pattje WJ, Schuuring E, Mastik MF, Slagter-Menkema L, Schrijvers ML, Alessi S, et al. The phosphatase and tensin homologue deleted on chromosome 10 mediates radiosensitivity in head and neck cancer. British journal of cancer. 2010;102(12):1778-85. Epub 2010/05/27.

[62] Pedrero JM, Carracedo DG, Pinto CM, Zapatero AH, Rodrigo JP, Nieto CS, et al. Frequent genetic and biochemical alterations of the PI 3-K/AKT/PTEN pathway in head and neck squamous cell carcinoma. International journal of cancer/Journal international du cancer. 2005;114(2):242-8. Epub 2004/11/16.

[63] Terakado N, Shintani S, Yano J, Chunnan L, Mihara M, Nakashiro K, et al. Overexpression of cyclooxygenase-2 is associated with radioresistance in oral squamous cell carcinoma. Oral oncology. 2004;40(4):383-9. Epub 2004/02/19.

[64] Freudlsperger C, Horn D, Weissfuss S, Weichert W, Weber KJ, Saure D, et al. Phosphorylation of AKT(Ser473) serves as an independent prognostic marker for radiosensitivity in advanced head and neck squamous cell carcinoma. International journal of cancer/Journal international du cancer. 2014. Epub 2014/11/13.

[65] Hassan KA, Ang KK, El-Naggar AK, Story MD, Lee JI, Liu D, et al. Cyclin B1 overexpression and resistance to radiotherapy in head and neck squamous cell carcinoma. Cancer research. 2002;62(22):6414-7. Epub 2002/11/20.

[66] Hassan KA, El-Naggar AK, Soria JC, Liu D, Hong WK, Mao L. Clinical significance of cyclin B1 protein expression in squamous cell carcinoma of the tongue. Clinical cancer research : an official journal of the American Association for Cancer Research. 2001;7(8):2458-62. Epub 2001/08/08.

[67] Akervall J, Nandalur S, Zhang J, Qian CN, Goldstein N, Gyllerup P, et al. A novel panel of biomarkers predicts radioresistance in patients with squamous cell carcinoma of the head and neck. Eur J Cancer. 2014;50(3):570-81. Epub 2013/12/18.

[68] Skvortsov S, Jimenez CR, Knol JC, Eichberger P, Schiestl B, Debbage P, et al. Radioresistant head and neck squamous cell carcinoma cells: intracellular signaling, putative biomarkers for tumor recurrences and possible therapeutic targets. Radiotherapy and oncology : journal of the European Society for Therapeutic Radiology and Oncology. 2011;101(1):177-82. Epub 2011/06/28.

[69] Skvortsov S, Dudas J, Eichberger P, Witsch-Baumgartner M, Loeffler-Ragg J, Pritz C, et al. Rac1 as a potential therapeutic target for chemo-radioresistant head and neck squamous cell carcinomas (HNSCC). British journal of cancer. 2014;110(11):2677-87. Epub 2014/05/03.

[70] Fukusumi T, Ishii H, Konno M, Yasui T, Nakahara S, Takenaka Y, et al. CD10 as a novel marker of therapeutic resistance and cancer stem cells in head and neck squamous cell carcinoma. British journal of cancer. 2014;111(3):506-14. Epub 2014/05/31.

[71] Eckers JC, Kalen AL, Sarsour EH, Tompkins VS, Janz S, Son JM, et al. Forkhead box M1 regulates quiescence-associated radioresistance of human head and neck squamous carcinoma cells. Radiation research. 2014;182(4):420-9. Epub 2014/09/18.

[72] Eschrich SA, Pramana J, Zhang H, Zhao H, Boulware D, Lee JH, et al. A gene expression model of intrinsic tumor radiosensitivity: prediction of response and prognosis after chemoradiation. International journal of radiation oncology, biology, physics. 2009;75(2):489-96. Epub 2009/09/09.

[73] Nana-Sinkam SP, Croce CM. MicroRNA dysregulation in cancer: opportunities for the development of microRNA-based drugs. IDrugs : the investigational drugs journal. 2010;13(12):843-6. Epub 2010/12/15.

[74] Babu JM, Prathibha R, Jijith VS, Hariharan R, Pillai MR. A miR-centric view of head and neck cancers. Biochimica et biophysica acta. 2011;1816(1):67-72. Epub 2011/05/10.

[75] Shiiba M, Uzawa K, Tanzawa H. MicroRNAs in Head and Neck Squamous Cell Carcinoma (HNSCC) and Oral Squamous Cell Carcinoma (OSCC). Cancers. 2010;2(2): 653-69. Epub 2010/01/01.

[76] Niemoeller OM, Niyazi M, Corradini S, Zehentmayr F, Li M, Lauber K, et al. MicroRNA expression profiles in human cancer cells after ionizing radiation. Radiat Oncol. 2011;6:29. Epub 2011/04/02.

[77] Childs G, Fazzari M, Kung G, Kawachi N, Brandwein-Gensler M, McLemore M, et al. Low-level expression of microRNAs let-7d and miR-205 are prognostic markers of

head and neck squamous cell carcinoma. The American journal of pathology. 2009;174(3):736-45. Epub 2009/01/31.

[78] Fletcher AM, Heaford AC, Trask DK. Detection of metastatic head and neck squamous cell carcinoma using the relative expression of tissue-specific mir-205. Translational oncology. 2008;1(4):202-8. Epub 2008/12/02.

[79] Hui AB, Lenarduzzi M, Krushel T, Waldron L, Pintilie M, Shi W, et al. Comprehensive MicroRNA profiling for head and neck squamous cell carcinomas. Clinical cancer research : an official journal of the American Association for Cancer Research. 2010;16(4):1129-39. Epub 2010/02/11.

[80] Shiiba M, Shinozuka K, Saito K, Fushimi K, Kasamatsu A, Ogawara K, et al. MicroRNA-125b regulates proliferation and radioresistance of oral squamous cell carcinoma. British journal of cancer. 2013;108(9):1817-21. Epub 2013/04/18.

[81] Wu SY, Lin KC, Chiou JF, Jeng SC, Cheng WH, Chang CI, et al. MicroRNA-17-5p post-transcriptionally regulates p21 expression in irradiated betel quid chewing-related oral squamous cell carcinoma cells. Strahlentherapie und Onkologie : Organ der Deutschen Rontgengesellschaft [et al]. 2013;189(8):675-83. Epub 2013/06/20.

[82] Summerer I, Niyazi M, Unger K, Pitea A, Zangen V, Hess J, et al. Changes in circulating microRNAs after radiochemotherapy in head and neck cancer patients. Radiat Oncol. 2013;8:296. Epub 2014/01/01.

[83] Vissink A, Jansma J, Spijkervet FK, Burlage FR, Coppes RP. Oral sequelae of head and neck radiotherapy. Critical reviews in oral biology and medicine : an official publication of the American Association of Oral Biologists. 2003;14(3):199-212. Epub 2003/06/12.

[84] Thorn JJ, Hansen HS, Specht L, Bastholt L. Osteoradionecrosis of the jaws: clinical characteristics and relation to the field of irradiation. Journal of oral and maxillofacial surgery : official journal of the American Association of Oral and Maxillofacial Surgeons. 2000;58(10):1088-93; discussion 93-5. Epub 2000/10/06.

[85] Overgaard J, Hansen HS, Specht L, Overgaard M, Grau C, Andersen E, et al. Five compared with six fractions per week of conventional radiotherapy of squamous-cell carcinoma of head and neck: DAHANCA 6 and 7 randomised controlled trial. Lancet. 2003;362(9388):933-40. Epub 2003/09/27.

[86] Du Y, Peyser ND, Grandis JR. Integration of molecular targeted therapy with radiation in head and neck cancer. Pharmacology & therapeutics. 2014;142(1):88-98. Epub 2013/11/28.

[87] Petrelli F, Coinu A, Riboldi V, Borgonovo K, Ghilardi M, Cabiddu M, et al. Concomitant platinum-based chemotherapy or cetuximab with radiotherapy for locally advanced head and neck cancer: A systematic review and meta-analysis of published studies. Oral oncology. 2014;50(11):1041-8. Epub 2014/09/02.

[88] Hama T, Yuza Y, Saito Y, J Ou, Kondo S, Okabe M, et al. Prognostic significance of epidermal growth factor receptor phosphorylation and mutation in head and neck squamous cell carcinoma. The oncologist. 2009;14(9):900-8. Epub 2009/09/04.

[89] Vermorken JB, Stohlmacher-Williams J, Davidenko I, Licitra L, Winquist E, Villanueva C, et al. Cisplatin and fluorouracil with or without panitumumab in patients with recurrent or metastatic squamous-cell carcinoma of the head and neck (SPECTRUM): an open-label phase 3 randomised trial. The lancet oncology. 2013;14(8):697-710. Epub 2013/06/12.

[90] Gonzalez JE, Barquinero JF, Lee M, Garcia O, Casaco A. Radiosensitization induced by the anti-epidermal growth factor receptor monoclonal antibodies cetuximab and nimotuzumab in A431 cells. Cancer biology & therapy. 2012;13(2):71-6. Epub 2012/01/11.

[91] Huang SM, Li J, Armstrong EA, Harari PM. Modulation of radiation response and tumor-induced angiogenesis after epidermal growth factor receptor inhibition by ZD1839 (Iressa). Cancer research. 2002;62(15):4300-6. Epub 2002/08/03.

[92] Bozec A, Sudaka A, Fischel JL, Brunstein MC, Etienne-Grimaldi MC, Milano G. Combined effects of bevacizumab with erlotinib and irradiation: a preclinical study on a head and neck cancer orthotopic model. British journal of cancer. 2008;99(1):93-9. Epub 2008/06/26.

[93] Chinnaiyan P, Huang S, Vallabhaneni G, Armstrong E, Varambally S, Tomlins SA, et al. Mechanisms of enhanced radiation response following epidermal growth factor receptor signaling inhibition by erlotinib (Tarceva). Cancer research. 2005;65(8): 3328-35. Epub 2005/04/19.

[94] Gustafson DL, Frederick B, Merz AL, Raben D. Dose scheduling of the dual VEGFR and EGFR tyrosine kinase inhibitor vandetanib (ZD6474, Zactima) in combination with radiotherapy in EGFR-positive and EGFR-null human head and neck tumor xenografts. Cancer chemotherapy and pharmacology. 2008;61(2):179-88. Epub 2007/03/30.

[95] Sano D, Matsumoto F, Valdecanas DR, Zhao M, Molkentine DP, Takahashi Y, et al. Vandetanib restores head and neck squamous cell carcinoma cells' sensitivity to cisplatin and radiation in vivo and in vitro. Clinical cancer research : an official journal of the American Association for Cancer Research. 2011;17(7):1815-27. Epub 2011/02/26.

[96] Bozec A, Sudaka A, Toussan N, Fischel JL, Etienne-Grimaldi MC, Milano G. Combination of sunitinib, cetuximab and irradiation in an orthotopic head and neck cancer model. Annals of oncology : official journal of the European Society for Medical Oncology / ESMO. 2009;20(10):1703-7. Epub 2009/06/23.

[97] Yadav A, Kumar B, Teknos TN, Kumar P. Sorafenib enhances the antitumor effects of chemoradiation treatment by downregulating ERCC-1 and XRCC-1 DNA repair proteins. Molecular cancer therapeutics. 2011;10(7):1241-51. Epub 2011/05/10.

[98] Li C, Iida M, Dunn EF, Wheeler DL. Dasatinib blocks cetuximab- and radiation-induced nuclear translocation of the epidermal growth factor receptor in head and neck squamous cell carcinoma. Radiotherapy and oncology : journal of the European Society for Therapeutic Radiology and Oncology. 2010;97(2):330-7. Epub 2010/07/30.

[99] Raju U, Riesterer O, Wang ZQ, Molkentine DP, Molkentine JM, Johnson FM, et al. Dasatinib, a multi-kinase inhibitor increased radiation sensitivity by interfering with nuclear localization of epidermal growth factor receptor and by blocking DNA repair pathways. Radiotherapy and oncology : journal of the European Society for Therapeutic Radiology and Oncology. 2012;105(2):241-9. Epub 2012/09/27.

[100] Tamatani T, Takamaru N, Hara K, Kinouchi M, Kuribayashi N, Ohe G, et al. Bortezomib-enhanced radiosensitization through the suppression of radiation-induced nuclear factor-kappaB activity in human oral cancer cells. International journal of oncology. 2013;42(3):935-44. Epub 2013/01/24.

[101] Weber CN, Cerniglia GJ, Maity A, Gupta AK. Bortezomib sensitizes human head and neck carcinoma cells SQ20B to radiation. Cancer biology & therapy. 2007;6(2):156-9. Epub 2007/01/17.

[102] Fujita T, Doihara H, Washio K, Kawasaki K, Takabatake D, Takahashi H, et al. Proteasome inhibitor bortezomib increases PTEN expression and enhances trastuzumab-induced growth inhibition in trastuzumab-resistant cells. Anti-cancer drugs. 2006;17(4):455-62. Epub 2006/03/22.

[103] Fu S, Rivera M, Ko EC, Sikora AG, Chen CT, Vu HL, et al. Combined inhibition of epidermal growth factor receptor and cyclooxygenase-2 as a novel approach to enhance radiotherapy. Journal of cell science & therapy. 2011;1(2). Epub 2011/10/13.

[104] Cerniglia GJ, Karar J, Tyagi S, Christofidou-Solomidou M, Rengan R, Koumenis C, et al. Inhibition of autophagy as a strategy to augment radiosensitization by the dual phosphatidylinositol 3-kinase/mammalian target of rapamycin inhibitor NVP-BEZ235. Molecular pharmacology. 2012;82(6):1230-40. Epub 2012/09/20.

[105] Gurtner K, Hessel F, Eicheler W, Dorfler A, Zips D, Heider KH, et al. Combined treatment of the immunoconjugate bivatuzumab mertansine and fractionated irradiation improves local tumour control in vivo. Radiotherapy and oncology : journal of the European Society for Therapeutic Radiology and Oncology. 2012;102(3):444-9. Epub 2011/11/22.

[106] Bauman JE, Ferris RL. Integrating novel therapeutic monoclonal antibodies into the management of head and neck cancer. Cancer. 2014;120(5):624-32. Epub 2013/11/14.

[107] Strano S, Dell'Orso S, Mongiovi AM, Monti O, Lapi E, Di Agostino S, et al. Mutant p53 proteins: between loss and gain of function. Head & neck. 2007;29(5):488-96. Epub 2006/11/24.

[108] Tassone P, Old M, Teknos TN, Pan Q. p53-based therapeutics for head and neck squamous cell carcinoma. Oral oncology. 2013;49(8):733-7. Epub 2013/04/30.

[109] Liu TJ, el-Naggar AK, McDonnell TJ, Steck KD, Wang M, Taylor DL, et al. Apoptosis induction mediated by wild-type p53 adenoviral gene transfer in squamous cell carcinoma of the head and neck. Cancer research. 1995;55(14):3117-22. Epub 1995/07/15.

[110] Pirollo KF, Hao Z, Rait A, Jang YJ, Fee WE, Jr., Ryan P, et al. p53 mediated sensitization of squamous cell carcinoma of the head and neck to radiotherapy. Oncogene. 1997;14(14):1735-46. Epub 1997/04/10.

[111] Clayman GL, el-Naggar AK, Lippman SM, Henderson YC, Frederick M, Merritt JA, et al. Adenovirus-mediated p53 gene transfer in patients with advanced recurrent head and neck squamous cell carcinoma. Journal of clinical oncology : official journal of the American Society of Clinical Oncology. 1998;16(6):2221-32. Epub 1998/06/17.

[112] Yoo GH, Moon J, Leblanc M, Lonardo F, Urba S, Kim H, et al. A phase 2 trial of surgery with perioperative INGN 201 (Ad5CMV-p53) gene therapy followed by chemoradiotherapy for advanced, resectable squamous cell carcinoma of the oral cavity, oropharynx, hypopharynx, and larynx: report of the Southwest Oncology Group. Archives of otolaryngology--head & neck surgery. 2009;135(9):869-74. Epub 2009/09/23.

[113] Nemunaitis J. Head and neck cancer: response to p53-based therapeutics. Head & neck. 2011;33(1):131-4. Epub 2010/03/12.

[114] Pearson S, Jia H, Kandachi K. China approves first gene therapy. Nature biotechnology. 2004;22(1):3-4. Epub 2004/01/06.

[115] Khuri FR, Nemunaitis J, Ganly I, Arseneau J, Tannock IF, Romel L, et al. a controlled trial of intratumoral ONYX-015, a selectively-replicating adenovirus, in combination with cisplatin and 5-fluorouracil in patients with recurrent head and neck cancer. Nature medicine. 2000;6(8):879-85. Epub 2000/08/10.

[116] Yuki K, Takahashi A, Ota I, Ohnishi K, Yasumoto J, Kanata H, et al. Glycerol enhances CDDP-induced growth inhibition of thyroid anaplastic carcinoma tumor carrying mutated p53 gene. Oncology reports. 2004;11(4):821-4. Epub 2004/03/11.

[117] Roh JL, Kang SK, Minn I, Califano JA, Sidransky D, Koch WM. p53-Reactivating small molecules induce apoptosis and enhance chemotherapeutic cytotoxicity in head and neck squamous cell carcinoma. Oral oncology. 2011;47(1):8-15. Epub 2010/11/27.

[118] Hummel R, Hussey DJ, Haier J. MicroRNAs: predictors and modifiers of chemo- and radiotherapy in different tumour types. Eur J Cancer. 2010;46(2):298-311. Epub 2009/12/02.

[119] Courthod G, Franco P, Palermo L, Pisconti S, Numico G. The role of microRNA in head and neck cancer: current knowledge and perspectives. Molecules. 2014;19(5): 5704-16. Epub 2014/05/08.

[120] Janssen HL, Reesink HW, Lawitz EJ, Zeuzem S, Rodriguez-Torres M, Patel K, et al. Treatment of HCV infection by targeting microRNA. The New England journal of medicine. 2013;368(18):1685-94. Epub 2013/03/29.

[121] Janiszewska J, Szaumkessel M, Szyfter K. microRNAs are important players in head and neck carcinoma: a review. Critical reviews in oncology/hematology. 2013;88(3): 716-28. Epub 2013/08/21.

[122] Juo P, Woo MS, Kuo CJ, Signorelli P, Biemann HP, Hannun YA, et al. FADD is required for multiple signaling events downstream of the receptor Fas. Cell growth & differentiation : the molecular biology journal of the American Association for Cancer Research. 1999;10(12):797-804. Epub 2000/01/05.

[123] Kruyt FA. TRAIL and cancer therapy. Cancer letters. 2008;263(1):14-25. Epub 2008/03/11.

[124] Walczak H, Miller RE, Ariail K, Gliniak B, Griffith TS, Kubin M, et al. Tumoricidal activity of tumor necrosis factor-related apoptosis-inducing ligand in vivo. Nature medicine. 1999;5(2):157-63. Epub 1999/02/04.

[125] Chen DJ, Huerta S. Smac mimetics as new cancer therapeutics. Anti-cancer drugs. 2009;20(8):646-58. Epub 2009/06/25.

[126] Du C, Fang M, Li Y, Li L, Wang X. Smac, a mitochondrial protein that promotes cytochrome c-dependent caspase activation by eliminating IAP inhibition. Cell. 2000;102(1):33-42. Epub 2000/08/10.

[127] Gasparini C, Vecchi Brumatti L, Monasta L, Zauli G. TRAIL-based therapeutic approaches for the treatment of pediatric malignancies. Current medicinal chemistry. 2013;20(17):2254-71. Epub 2013/03/06.

[128] Raulf N, El-Attar R, Kulms D, Lecis D, Delia D, Walczak H, et al. Differential response of head and neck cancer cell lines to TRAIL or Smac mimetics is associated with the cellular levels and activity of caspase-8 and caspase-10. British journal of cancer. 2014;111(10):1955-64. Epub 2014/10/15.

[129] Kumar B, Yadav A, Hideg K, Kuppusamy P, Teknos TN, Kumar P. A novel curcumin analog (H-4073) enhances the therapeutic efficacy of cisplatin treatment in head and neck cancer. PloS one. 2014;9(3):e93208. Epub 2014/03/29.

[130] Tuttle S, Hertan L, Daurio N, Porter S, Kaushick C, Li D, et al. The chemopreventive and clinically used agent curcumin sensitizes HPV (-) but not HPV (+) HNSCC to ionizing radiation, in vitro and in a mouse orthotopic model. Cancer biology & therapy. 2012;13(7):575-84. Epub 2012/03/24.

[131] Masuelli L, Di Stefano E, Fantini M, Mattera R, Benvenuto M, Marzocchella L, et al. Resveratrol potentiates the in vitro and in vivo anti-tumoral effects of curcumin in head and neck carcinomas. Oncotarget. 2014;5(21):10745-62. Epub 2014/10/10.

[132] Deng R, Wang X, Liu Y, Yan M, Hanada S, Xu Q, et al. A new gamboge derivative compound 2 inhibits cancer stem-like cells via suppressing EGFR tyrosine phosphorylation in head and neck squamous cell carcinoma. Journal of cellular and molecular medicine. 2013;17(11):1422-33. Epub 2013/10/12.

Chapter 2

The Six Rs of Head and Neck Cancer Radiotherapy

Loredana G. Marcu, Iuliana Toma Dasu and Alexandru Dasu

Additional information is available at the end of the chapter

http://dx.doi.org/10.5772/60015

1. Introduction

Locally advanced head and neck cancers are usually aggressive tumours, due to the presence of hypoxia and the ability of the tumour to repopulate during treatment. The aggressive behaviour generally requires aggressive treatment, which for head and neck carcinomas consist of altered radiotherapy fractionation schedules combined with chemotherapy. Treatment fractionation, based on the 4 Rs of radiotherapy [1] is a well-accepted concept that has been re-adjusted for head and neck cancer decades ago to accommodate new radiobiological findings. The 4 Rs in terms of *repair, repopulation, reoxygenation, and redistribution* along the cell cycle have been promoted to 5 Rs with the aid of *radiosensitivity* and more recently to 6 Rs with the experimental evidence of *remote* (bystander) *cellular effects*.

The paragaphs below aim to describe the major aspects concerning the six Rs of radiotherapy applied to head and neck cancer.

2. The 5 Rs revisited

The 5 Rs of radiobiology represent a group of processes determining the response of cells and tissues to radiation, with great impact in fractionated irradiation. Balancing them one against the other has become one of the pillars of modern radiation therapy to maximise the therapeutic gain by either increasing radiation damage in the tumour cells or decreasing the damage to the normal tissues. The impact of the individual Rs varies across the different tissues, but for head and neck tumours all of them play important roles that have to be taken into account when designing successful radiotherapy schedules.

2.1. Repair

Repair is a term covering a number of processes responsible for the identification and correction of the damage to the DNA molecule induced by endogenous and exogenous factors. Sometimes the term "recovery" is used instead of "repair" because other processes are involved besides the actual repair of damage. The importance of recovery or repair in relation to irradiation has been determined in a series of experiments employing continuous irradiation at various dose-rates or split-dose experiments studying the variation of the cell survival with irradiation time or the time between individual fractions of radiation. Following these types of experiments radiation damage has been divided into two categories, non-repairable or lethal damage and repairable or sublethal damage. It should be remarked that these are operational terms that have not been correlated with any type of radiation-induced damage, with the possible exception of the irreparable clusters of damage. Sublethal damage could be removed as part of the cell recovery, unless fixated by interaction with other sublethal lesions or by being forced to be expressed by the cells. Consequently, cell survival following irradiation depends not only on the creation of irreparable lesions, but also on the competition between repair and fixation of sublethal damage that is influenced by many factors including the rate of generating new lesions and the cellular environment.

When describing the effect of radiation with the help of the well-known cell survival curves, the repairable component of damage is considered responsible for the shoulder of the curve as the accumulation of damage in the absence of the repair increases cell kill. Consequently the recovery capacity of cells could be quantified by relating the "bendiness" of the cell survival curve to its initial slope that is a measure of the irreparable or lethal damage induced by radiation. For the linear-quadratic (LQ) model [2,3] this is given by the beta/alpha ratio, which is low for acutely reacting normal tissues and most tumours including head and neck tumours and high for late reacting tissues [4]. This indicates the high potential for recovery of late reacting tissue that should be exploited in head and neck radiotherapy to limit the late complication rates.

Several models have been proposed to account for the process of recovery, including the incomplete repair model [5], the lethal-potentially-lethal model [6] or the repairable-conditionally repairable damage model [7], with the incomplete repair model, based itself on the LQ formalism, being mostly known and employed in clinical practice. According to the incomplete repair model [5], the effect of continuous irradiation delivering radiation dose D in time t is given by equation 1.

$$E = \alpha \dot{d} t + g(t)\beta(\dot{d} t)^2 \tag{1}$$

where α and β are parameters of the LQ model and g is a function describing the repair taking place in time t. If the repair is described as an exponential process, with repair constant μ, the g term is described by the expression in equation 2.

$$g(\mu t) = 2\frac{[\mu t - 1 + exp(-\mu t)]}{(\mu t)^2} \tag{2}$$

http://dx.doi.org/10.5772/60015

Similar expressions could be derived for the case of fractionated irradiation, when the focus is on the repair taking place between the individual fractions. Thus, the effect in fractionated radiation with time t between fractions is given by the expression in equation 3.

$$E = n\left[\alpha d + h\left(t\right)\beta d^{2}\right] \tag{3}$$

where n is the number of fractions, d is the dose per fraction and the repair term $h(t)$ is given by the expression in equation 4.

$$h\left(t\right) = \frac{2}{n}\frac{exp(-\mu t)}{1 - exp(-\mu t)}\left[n - \frac{1 - exp(-n\mu t)}{1 - exp(-\mu t)}\right] \tag{4}$$

These expressions could be used together with the Biological Effective Dose (BED) formalism [8,9] to calculate the effectiveness of various treatment approaches. Thus, the expressions in equations 1 and 2 are mostly suited for brachytherapy, while expressions in equations 3 and 4 are suited for fractionated therapy when intra-fraction repair is considered negligible. Expressions have also been derived to account simultaneously for intra and inter-fraction repair [10].

A number of studies have determined relevant repair constants from clinical and experimental data, yielding values between 0.5 and 2 h for the repair half-life, depending on the tissue and the type of experiment used to derive them [11]. More recent studies indicated that the rate of repair might depend on the dose or that second order or bi- or even multi-exponential processes might exist [12-15]. The multi-exponential processes appear to be equally divided between the fast and the slow components with median repair half-lives of 0.3 h for the fast component and about 4 h for the slow component (for a summary see [16]). In this context it has been pointed out that identification of the relevant rates might depend on the design of the experiment as it has been suggested that split-dose experiments could easily miss a fast component of repair [16].

Repair or recovery of radiation damage has been extensively exploited to spare late reacting normal tissues in head and neck radiation therapy. Thus, the low alpha/beta ratio (or high beta/alpha ratio) of these tissues in comparison to the tumours indicates their high capacity for repair in fractionated regimes if enough time is allowed between individual fractions for the recovery of sublethal damage. Consequently, decreasing the dose per fraction can protect late reacting normal tissues more than the tumour cells, this differential effect allowing an escalation of the dose to the tumours in comparison to conventional fractionation or a decrease in the expected complication rates to maximise the therapeutic gain. Indeed, several clinical studies initiated in the 1980s and 1990s have shown that increased fractionation in head and neck radiotherapy could increase the control rates for the same levels of complications or could even reduce the complication rates. Thus, Bourhis *et al* [17] performed a meta-analysis of hyperfractionated trials in head and neck cancer, and reported a significant benefit from hyperfractionation than with conventional fractionation on survival (8% at 5 years) and on locoregional control (6.4% at 5 years).

Hyperfractionated regimes employing very small fractions required that they are given twice or three times per day to keep the overall treatment times to manageable lengths that avoid problems from tumour repopulation (see section II.2). Some of these treatment schedules highlighted the clinical implications of not allowing enough time between fractions for complete recovery of sublethal damage. One of the most known examples is the Continuous Hyperfractionated Accelerated Radiotherapy (CHART) trial delivering 54 Gy in 36 fractions in 12 consecutive days [18]. While the trial demonstrated a similar level of local control with 66 Gy in 33 daily fractions for a significant reduction in late treatment-related morbidity, the reduction was much less than expected from BED calculations. Analyses of the complication rates in the conventional and hyperfractionated arms showed that the repair half-life might indeed be 4-5 h, which is quite long for the 6 h interfraction intervals in the hyperfractionated arm of CHART [19]. The high amount of residual damage after the slow component of recovery might also explain why twice daily fractionation schemes with 2 Gy per fraction sometimes led to too high rates of late effects [20]. Nevertheless, twice daily fractionation regimes employing 1.2 or even 1.6 Gy per fraction have been safely used for treatment [21-24] and illustrate how the differential recovery potential of late and acutely reacting tissue could be exploited to increase the therapeutic potential in the radiation therapy of head and neck cancers.

In fact the potential for improvement of any fractionation scheme employing n fractions of size d could be evaluated using the BED formalism. Thus, the biologically equivalent of total dose in 2 Gy fractions (EQD) could be derived for the effects in late reacting tissues using an alpha/beta ratio of 3 Gy (equation 5) and in tumours and acutely reacting tissues using an alpha/beta of 10 Gy (equation 6).

$$EQD_3 = nd\frac{1+\frac{d}{3}}{1+\frac{2}{3}} \tag{5}$$

$$EQD_{10} = nd\frac{1+\frac{d}{10}}{1+\frac{2}{10}} \tag{6}$$

where $1+\frac{2}{3}$ is the relative effectiveness of conventional fractionation regimes in late reacting tissues and $1+\frac{2}{10}$ is the relative effectiveness of conventional fractionation regimes in acutely reacting tissues and tumours. The expressions could be adapted to include the effect of incomplete recovery between fractions (equations 3 and 4) or for protracted irradiation (equations 1 and 2). In fact, the loss of effects due to protracted irradiation has been a cause of concern in some applications like intensity modulated radiotherapy (IMRT), although this loss might not be significant as long as the delivery time is shorter than the half-life of the quick component of recovery [16].

2.2. Repopulation

Besides repair, repopulation during treatment is another important factor that could modulate the response to fractionated regimes. Indeed, as the effects in radiotherapy are related to the inactivation of cells from tumours and normal tissues, any proliferative process taking place during treatment will increase the cell population and consequently diminish the effect of radiation therapy. The effect would therefore depend on the time available for proliferation, i.e., the overall treatment time, and will particularly be a problem for acutely reacting tissues and tumours that have significant proliferation. In late reacting tissues in contrast, proliferative activity is minimal during the few days or weeks required by most treatment schedules and the treatment duration will not influence the complication rates.

The existence of a time factor in clinical radiation therapy was recognised quite early and gave rise to the Strandquist plots [25] and the nominal standard dose (NSD) concept [26] attempting to relate the time, dose and fractionation of equivalent fractionation regimes. However, an important breakthrough linking the time factor to the proliferation of tumour cells was made following the publication by Withers and colleagues of a study analysing the total dose needed to achieve 50% control for squamous tumours of the head and neck as a function of the overall treatment time [27]. The results showed that there was an increase of the required dose at a rate of 0.5-0.6 Gy per day for treatments lasting more than about 21-28 days, which was attributed to accelerated proliferation taking place in tumours after the lag time. This report was accompanied by the development of the BED concept with proliferation [9]. Thus, the effect of proliferation with doubling time T_p for a treatment with n fractions of size d being delivered in time T could be accounted by equation 7

$$BED = nd\left[1 + \frac{d}{\alpha/\beta}\right] - \frac{\ln(2)}{\alpha T_p}\left(T - T_k\right) \quad (7)$$

where T_k is the delay in the onset of proliferation. The equation could be further adapted to include the effects of repair as described in equations 1-4.

A series of clinical studies have investigated the impact of overall treatment time and proliferation on the outcome of radiation therapy for head and neck tumours. Studies investigating only the impact of acceleration, i.e., the delivery of more than 10 Gy per week that is the norm in conventional fractionation delivered in 5 daily fractions per week, have reported better control, but also an increase in acute reactions and sometimes an increase in late reactions when the interfraction interval was too short to allow full repair of sublethal damage [20,28,29]. More successful were schedules combining hyperfractionation and acceleration by delivering two or more fractions per day [18,22,30,31]. Nevertheless, an analysis performed by Bourhis and colleagues found a small but statistically significant benefit of 2% on survival at 5 years from acceleration itself in comparison to conventional fractionation [17].

The overall treatment time analysis of head and neck tumours indicates proliferation doubling time of the order of 3 to 5 days. This corresponds to the values determined from measurements of the potential doubling time of tumours, T_{pot} [32]. Whether T_p in equation 7 is T_{pot} is still a matter of debate. Experimental studies have shown that the effective doubling time for proliferation during radiotherapy could be either smaller or larger than T_{pot} [33]. A large multicentre analysis also failed to correlate experimental determinations of T_{pot} with treatment outcome in head and neck cancers [34]. However, a more recent analysis has shown that pre-treatment proliferation parameters are better predictors of outcome when other factors like tumour size, individual radiosensitivity and overall treatment time are taken into account [35].

The increase in acute reactions when shortening the overall treatment time indicates that compensatory proliferation is also part of the mechanisms available for the rapidly proliferating normal tissues to recover from radiation damage. However, it has been found that the kinetic parameters for acute reactions are significantly different from those from tumours [36]. Thus, acute mucosal reactions that may become a limiting factor in the radiotherapy of head and neck tumours have a T_k of 7 days and a T_p of 2.5 days. This difference has given the opportunity to search for an optimum overall treatment time that maximises tumour effect, without jeopardising the function of late and acute normal tissues [37,38].

Three mechanisms have been proposed to be behind accelerated proliferation, namely asymmetry loss and acceleration of divisions of the stem cell compartment, as well as abortive divisions of sterilised cells [39]. Recruitment of quiescent cells into the cell cycle has also been proposed. The molecular triggers for these mechanisms remain to be elucidated [40], although there are some indications that epidermal growth factor receptor (EGFR) and protein tyrosine phosphatase (PTEN) activation might be involved [41-44].

Ample modelling of the aforementioned proliferation mechanisms has been undertaken in order to quantify the extent of repopulation during treatment, to study the individual contribution of each mechanism as well as their interplay towards overall tumour repopulation [45,46]. It was shown that while cell recruitment does contribute towards repopulation to a small extent, the major mechanism responsible for accelerated proliferation of tumour cells during radiotherapy is the asymmetry loss of stem cell division.

2.3. Reoxygenation

Tumour oxygenation is known to be one of the main factors that determine the response to radiotherapy. For advanced head and neck cancer in particular, clinical trials have shown that pre-treatment polarographic measurements of tumour oxygenation indicating the presence of tumour hypoxia correlate with poor prognosis [47]. This clinical evidence of the role of tumour hypoxia in determining the outcome of the treatment has been further confirmed by several studies in which pre-treatment uptake of nitroimidazole compounds such as ^{18}F-Fluoromisonidazole (^{18}F-MISO) or Cu-diacetyl-bis(N4-methylthiosemicarbazone) (Cu-ATSM) used as Positron Emission Tomography (PET) hypoxia imaging agents was shown to predict the outcome in head and neck cancer radiotherapy [48]. Furthermore, pre-treatment tumour hypoxia does not only correlate with poor local control due to the presence of resistant cells to radiotherapy, but also to chemotherapy and poor long time prognosis because of the loco-regional spread and formation of distant metastases [49].

The mechanism of resistance of tumour hypoxic cells to radiation can be explained by the so-called oxygen effect related to the oxygen actions at the level of the free radicals formed after the interaction of charged particles with biological material. The free radicals, which are highly reactive molecules because of their unpaired valence electron, are responsible for the break of the DNA chemical bonds which might be further made permanent by molecular oxygen. The resulting biological damage depends thus on the presence or absence of oxygen, well-oxygenated cells being more sensitive to radiation induced damage than hypoxic cells deprived of oxygen.

Given the clinically proven impact of the presence of hypoxia on the treatment outcome, it is important to investigate the mechanisms of the occurrence of tumour hypoxia and its dynamics. The impaired oxygen supply to tumour cells leading to the formation of tumour hypoxia originates in the particularities of the tumour vasculature formed mainly through parasitation of the normal tissue vasculature and angiogenesis. Consequently, the major mechanisms involved in the formation of hypoxia are related to either the actual architecture of the blood vessels and the diffusion-limited delivery of oxygen, or to the functional abnormalities of tumour capillaries leading to perfusion limitations [49]. The two main forms of hypoxia associated with them are known as chronic (diffusion-limited) or acute (perfusion-limited) hypoxia. Thus, chronic hypoxia will occur when the distance from the cells to the nearer capillaries is close to exceeding the maximum oxygen diffusion distance, which under normal rates of oxygen consumption by the cells is expected to be in the order of 100-150 μm as shown by the early studies of Thomlinson and Gray [50] and confirmed later by experimental and modelling studies [51-53]. Acute hypoxia arises near the blood vessels temporary occluded, and, by its nature, has a transient character, unless the blood vessels remain blocked a long time period, depriving the cells of oxygen beyond the limit for survival.

For head and neck squamous cell carcinomas (HNSCC) in particular, which appear to be formed from nonvascularized epithelium, relatively hypoxic under normal conditions, hypoxia might pose particular reasons of concern. Thus, heterogeneous distributions of oxygen throughout the cellular microenvironment are expected in HNSCC. The impairment in the oxygen supply is not only spatially but also temporally heterogeneous.

Regardless the mechanism through which hypoxia occurs in tumours, there is a general consensus correlated to the clinical evidence that hypoxia is a negative predictive factor for the treatment and that patients might benefit from treatment strategies adapted according to the oxygenation of their individual tumours. However, it has also been suggested that chronically and acutely hypoxic cells might respond differently to radiation on the grounds of their energy supply and viability. It is well known that the combined high rate of glycolytic metabolism and poor availability of glucose result in low energy reserves for tumour cells reflected by the relative levels of ATP, ADP, AMP, Pi and PCr [54, 55]. The energy supply of chronically hypoxic cells, however, appears to decrease after a couple of hours of glucose deprivation [56] while the energy of well oxygenated cells does not decrease significantly under glucose deprivation. Therefore, one could postulate that chronically hypoxic cells are less capable to activate their DNA repair mechanisms and therefore would be more radiation sensitive compared to the acutely hypoxic cell [57] and quote in support studies on nutrient deprived cells [58,59]. Consequently, particular attention has to be paid to the cells at intermediate oxygen levels which might possess a dangerous combination of viability and partial radioresistance that might in turn be reflected in the poor outcome to radiation treatment [60,61].

The oxygen status of the tumour cells is however not static with respect to both spatial and temporal patterns. Changes in the cellular oxygenation related to the dynamics of both chronic and acute hypoxia are generally known as tumour reoxygenation.

Reoxygenation manifests itself following two main patterns. Temporal heterogeneity in oxygenation arises in relation to acute or perfusion-limited hypoxia. Abnormal vasculature can lead to fluctuations in the blood flow due to the temporary occlusion or even backflow. These phenomena have a rather chaotic but transient character and are conventionally referred to as fast reoxygenation [62] although in some cases the change in oxygen supply might in fact be from poor to well and back to poor, thus not necessarily leading to an improvement of the oxygenation of the cells but rather to a re-hypoxiation. The temporal scale of changes in oxygenation related to acute, perfusion limited hypoxia, ranges from minutes to hours as demonstrated by several experiments using sequential injection of different fluorescent dyes for hypoxia and vascular perfusion [63,64]. Furthermore, in presence of irradiation, the dynamics of the oxygenation might be even more pronounced as shown in a study on human laryngeal squamous cell carcinoma tumour line grown as xenografts in nude mice by Bussink *et al* [51] indicating that irradiation could lead to rapid changes in oxygenation and perfusion. Chronically hypoxic cells might also change their oxygenation status during the course of fractionated therapy through the so-called slow reoxygenation. In a mixed tumour cell population with respect to oxygenation, ionizing radiation will primarily kill the sensitive well-oxygenated cells. This would result in lower oxygen consumption and hence to larger distances of oxygen diffusion which independently or in conjunction to overall tumour shrinkage might lead to the improvement of the tumour oxygenation by reoxygenation of the chronically hypoxic cells. Furthermore, during long, fractionated, radiotherapy treatments, extending over several weeks, revascularisation of the tumour through angiogenesis might also occur resulting in the reoxygenation of cells that were chronically hypoxic.

Taking advantage of the changes in tumour oxygenation and expecting that they will result in an improvement of radiosensitivity by fractionating the dose and thus increasing the treatment duration is one of the first approaches clinically used for overcoming tumour hypoxia. However, the search for the optimal dose per fraction and number of fractions in which the treatment has to be delivered is far from being over considering that one has to find the right balance between the fractional dose that might overcome hypoxia and the number of fractions that will ensure proper reoxygenation accounting at the same time for the normal tissue and organs at risk.

There are several clinical studies indicating that the oxygenation of head and neck tumours is indeed dynamic. The early studies of changes in tumour oxygenation in advanced head and neck carcinoma using polarographic electrodes were inconclusive in proving that reoxygenation positively correlates to increased local control most likely due to the inherent limitations of the technique [65-67]. More recent studies, however, using PET imaging, started to shed more light on the clinical evidence of oxygenation changes and reoxygenation in head and neck tumours [68-70]. The general consensus is that hypoxic subvolumes identified with the use of PET imaging in head and neck cancer are inversely correlated with the response to radiotherapy and generally with the treatment outcome. The improvement in the tumour oxygenation together with the observed geometrical stability of the persistent hypoxic regions during the course of radiotherapy suggest that head and neck tumours are strong candidates for treatment strategies accounting for tumour hypoxia at the time of treatment planning and/ or treatment adaptation based on hypoxia PET imaging.

Clinical implementation of hypoxia-driven radiotherapy is, however, still in its infancy. Several strategies for dose-painting approaches based on hypoxia in head and neck tumours have been proposed and they are under various stages of validation. Among them one could mention the planning study by Thorwarth *et al* [71] on dose escalation to head and neck hypoxic subvolumes based on PET imaging which was followed by a still ongoing clinical trial and the dose prescription and treatment planning method based on hypoxia PET imaging proposed by Toma-Dasu *et al* [72] which is currently under clinical validation.

In addition to dose escalation, treatment strategies focusing on overcoming hypoxia could include radiosensitizers or hypoxic cytotoxins. Lin and Hahn [48] presented a conceptual multimodal adaptive clinical trial approach focusing on radiation dose escalation to hypoxic regions highlighting the importance of pretreatment hypoxia imaging in order to properly select the patients that would be expected to benefit from hypoxia targeted treatments. They envisaged that serial imaging should be performed during therapy to evaluate treatment response and to select in a step-wise manner the highest-risk areas warranting treatment modifications, such as radiation dose escalation and to select the candidates for radiosensitizers.

A special class of strategy in the management of advanced head and neck is represented by the anti-angiogenic treatment which addresses the vascular endothelial growth factors and their respective receptors on endothelial cells as well as their role in role in promoting the growth and progression of carcinoma of the head and neck. Several anti-angiogenic treatments have shown promising results in the clinical setting such as those using tyrosine kinase inhibitors or bevacizumab [73]. Nevertheless, the current results suggest that multimodal therapies combining anti-angiogenic agents with chemo/radiotherapy have the potential to further increase the overall clinical benefit.

2.4. Redistribution

Similar to other tumour cell populations, squamous cell carcinomas of the head and neck proliferate in asynchronous growth. Therefore cells will be distributed unevenly through the cell cycle phases. Yet, the most probable distribution is the exponential one, with the largest population in G1 and smallest in mitosis. Partial synchronisation can occur as a result of cell arrest in one or more cycle phases due to the effect of radiotherapy or chemotherapy.

Cellular redistribution or reassortment along the cell cycle plays an important role in the success of fractionated radiotherapy, given that cells present various radiosensitivities along the four phases of the cell cycle. Given the relatively short average cell cycle time of squamous cell carcinomas (around 33 hours) [62], cells that survive a first dose of radiation will tend to be in a resistant phase however, within a few hours they may progress into a more sensitive phase where they can be hit by radiation and killed.

Cells situated in the S phase are known to be about three times more radioresistant than cells undergoing mitosis. Since the duration of the S phase is about one third of the cell cycle length, there are large numbers of cells escaping the effect of radiation during a single hit. Fractionated radiotherapy assists in overcoming this challenge due to cellular redistribution between two consecutive doses.

Head and neck tumour cells have a high cell turnover, thus a relatively short cell cycle time. Cellular redistribution along the cell cycle for rapidly proliferating tumours consents to a more uniform cell kill than in slowly growing tumours. This rationale justifies the implementation of hyperfractionated radiotherapy schedules in head and neck cancers, which also hinders tumour repopulation during treatment.

Cells in the quiescent phase also play an important role during treatment as they can be triggered back into the cycle by cell loss due to radio- or chemotherapy. Quiescent cells are usually more resistant to radiation than cycling cells, fact that makes cellular recruitment (i.e. the process whereby quiescent cells re-enter the cell cycle) a double-edged sword: once they reach mitosis, newly cycling cells can increase the pool of tumour cells via cell division and, at the same time, cell killing can be more effective among cycling cells (as compared to quiescent cells) due to an overall higher radiosensitivity.

One of the known risk factors in head and neck cancer is the infection with HPV (human papillomavirus). A large number of studies have proven that head and neck cancers that are positive for HPV have higher cellular radiosensitivity than their non-HPV counterparts [74,75]. One of the explanations for this behaviour is the impaired DNA repair ability found among HPV-positive tumours and a considerable G_2 arrest. These experimental studies have shown that irradiated HPV-positive cells progress faster through the S phase and then accrue in G_2/M [75]. This unusual behaviour alters the expected cellular distribution along the cell cycle, accumulating the HPV cells in the more radiosensitive phases. Therefore, patients that tested positive for HPV respond better to the effect of radiotherapy and have a more favourable prognosis than non-HPV patients [74].

2.5. Radiosensitivity

Radiosensitivity is the tumour feature which aims to account for the fact that tumours respond differently to radiation therapy in a manner correlated with the intrinsic radiosensitivity of the cells derived as derived from *in vitro* experiments.

The intrinsic radiosensitivity influences the overall response of tumours to (chemo-) radiotherapy. The origins of the intrinsic radiosensitivity are related to the genetic instability of individual tumours leading to variations in response even among tumours of the same histological type [76]. Therefore, identifying *a priori* the alterations in the intracellular pathways involved in the DNA response, regulation of cell cycle and cell proliferation or responsible for activating the apoptotic signal, might offer the possibility of identifying the patients expected to respond poorly to radiation therapy due to intrinsic radioresistance and customising the treatment based on individual radiobiological and genetic features of the tumours.

The most often mentioned pathways that were identified as clinically relevant in relation to the intrinsic radiosensitivity are the activation of Epidermal Growth Factor Receptor (EGFR), p53 and Ki-67 proteins signalling cascades.

For head and neck in particular, the activation of the phosphatidylinositol-3-kinase (PI3-K)/ protein kinase B (AKT) pathway has been shown to be associated not only with intrinsic radioresistance but also with other well-known tumour features responsible to poor outcome, cell proliferation and tumour hypoxia. This is because the PI3-K/AKT is a key element for the regulation of several cellular processes like apoptosis, invasion and proliferation. Consequently, it has been proposed that the manipulation of this signal-transduction pathway could be used in the management of head and neck cancers. Given the activation of this pathway by the stimulation of receptor tyrosine kinases like the EGFR, it has been suggested that markers for PI3-K/AKT activation should be related to predictors of EGFR sensitivity. Furthermore, inhibiting the PI3-K/AKT pathway will antagonise radiation-induced cellular defence mechanisms that in turn will result in enhancing the effectiveness of radiation therapy [77].

More recently, a biomarker that encodes the p53 protein, TP53, has been identified as the most commonly altered gene in squamous cell carcinomas of the head and neck leading to radioresistance [78].

As already mentioned above, the presence of Human Papilloma Virus (HPV) influences the response of the response to radiotherapy for head and neck squamous cell carcinoma [79]. Thus, the HPV status of the tumour could be regarded as a strong and independent prognostic factor for the success of the treatment, both in terms of local regional control and overall survival. This is due the increased cellular radiosensitivity caused by compromised DNA repair capacity in HPV-positive cells [74]. This might indicate that radiosensitivity and repair in cells should be correlated. Two main mechanisms have been identified for the repair of the double strand breaks of the DNA, homologous recombination (HR) and nonhomologous end-joining (NHEJ). Nevertheless, it has been shown that mutations in genes that impair HR often cause only modest or no radiation hypersensitivity. In contrast, mutations in NHEJ genes appear to lead to greater radiation hypersensitivity [80]. These complex relationships may in fact be the reason for difficulties in finding a correlation between repair and radiosensitivity [81] and why these are considered as two independent Rs in radiation biology.

3. The 6th R: Remote bystander effects

Remote cellular effects or bystander effects occur when non-irradiated cells that are located nearby irradiated cells undergo cellular damage similar to the irradiated cells. This experimental observation contradicts the formerly accepted theory of radiation-induced targeted cell kill [82]. While targeted cells can be killed by radiation, according to the bystander theory, non-targeted cells can also present signs of radiation damage that eventually kills the cell. This happens as a consequence of cellular communication when radiation-hit cells direct damage signals through gap junctions to the neighbouring non-targeted cells, which then act as being hit by radiation.

Bystander effects have been evidenced in both tumour and normal cells, which implies that such remote effects could have clinical implications. The finding that gamma-ray-induced bystander effects have influence on epithelial cells and not fibroblasts, suggested that tissue architecture and also cell communication play a significant role in this process [83]. Since squamous cell carcinomas originate from epithelial cells, the bystander effect becomes an important consideration in the treatment of head and neck tumours (table 1).

It is known that in normal tissues, gap junctions physiologically connect one cell to the adjacent one to enable the transmission of genetic signals between cells. Both metabolic cooperation between cells and the regulation of normal tissue homeostasis requires the involvement of gap junctions. This normal phenotype is usually lost during head and neck carcinogenesis. Although the complete function of gap junctions in head and neck neoplasms is not fully clarified, experimental studies demonstrate that gap-junctional intercellular communication (GJIC) could mediate apoptotic cell death in non-targeted squamous cell carcinoma adjacent to individually targeted squamous cell carcinomas of the head and neck [84].

Novel therapeutic methods like gene therapy are widely used to investigate bystander effects in cancers including head and neck. A number of viral vectors have been developed that are able to transfer genes to therapy of tumours known as gene transduction. The occurrence of a bystander effect after wild-type p53 gene transduction has been investigated for human squamous cell carcinomas of the head and neck [85]. Wild-type p53 gene transduction for apoptosis-inducing molecular therapy has been shown capable of producing a bystander effect in squamous cells *in vitro*. Additionally, it was demonstrated that this phenomenon requires intercellular contact between wild-type p53 transduced and bystander, non-transduced cell populations. The study concluded that other therapies associated with apoptosis (such as radiotherapy or chemotherapy) might also demonstrate bystander effects.

Enhancing gap-junctional intercellular communication in squamous cell carcinomas of the head and neck and understanding the other mechanisms behind cancer cell communication may lead to increased therapeutic efficacy.

Bystander effect	Mode of cellular communication	Reference
Growth inhibition	Intercellular contact between wild-type p53 transduced and non-transduced cell population	Frank *et al* 1998 [85]
Apoptotic cell death		Frank *et al* 2005 [84]
Genomic instability	Cellular interaction influenced by stromal fibroblasts	Kamochi *et al* 2008 [86]
Cell dormancy and proliferation arrest	Gap-junctional intercellular communication	Kucerova *et al* 2013 [87]

Table 1. Bystander effects in squamous cell carcinoma of the head and neck

An interesting observation that could have implications in the development of new therapeutical agents for cancer was reported by Cogan *et al* [88]. The group has shown that bystander signals from cancer cells after exposure to chromium VI results in DNA damage in neighbouring cells that is strongly dependent on telomerase (complex enzyme that maintains the telomere length). Low dose exposure to Cr(VI) was able to induce cancer cells to continuously secrete bystander signals that caused DNA damage in the neighbouring cells. However, these bystander signals were telomerase-dependent, meaning that the status of the telomere (negative or positive) has dictated the affinity of cancer cells for bystander signals.

It is well known that telomere activation has a therapeutic potential for cancer, given that with each cell division, the length of telomeres shortens, fact that triggers cell senescence. In order to survive, cancer cells are required to employ a mechanism to stabilise this process of telomere reduction. There are several reports in the literature showing that telomerase promoter mutations (TERT) are more prevalent in aggressive cancers and they are a major indicator of poor prognosis among head and neck cancer patients [89,90]. The effect of chromium VI on telomerase offers, therefore, a potential anticancer avenue that needs to be further explored.

Bystander effects largely relate to nontargeted effects after exposure to low dose radiation. While tumours are targeted with high doses, the surrounding normal tissue receives much lower doses of radiation and organs that are out-of-field even lower doses. Exposure of nontargeted tissue raises several concerns regarding the risk of second primary cancers. However, it was shown that low dose exposure of healthy cells (2 - 50 mGy) stimulates intercellular induction of apoptosis in the precancerous cell population, via cytokine and reactive oxygen species signalling [91]. This selective elimination of precancerous cells could reduce the incidence of second cancers following radiotherapy.

There is a limited number of studies on the risk of second cancers after primary head and neck carcinoma treatment and they reveal the observation that among these patients second cancers occur, most often, due to smoking [92] and drinking habits [93]. Second cancers are common among long-term survivals, however they are not necessarily second primaries. Recurrences occur very often and they arise mostly in the treatment field [94]. Common sites for second primary cancers are the lung and the esophagus. These occurrences are often linked to the same risk factors as for the primary head and neck cancer, i.e. tobacco smoking and alcohol consumption. The radiation-induced incidence of second primary cancers after head and neck radiotherapy was analysed in a study by Yamamoto *et al* [95]. The group has concluded that radiotherapy of the primary tumour is not thought to be associated with an increased risk of second tumours. Furthermore, it was underlined that a clonal relationship exists between the primary head and neck cancer and second primaries, suggesting that the latter are a result of micrometastatic foci migration from the site of origin.

Beside bystander effects, there is another phenomenon that is linked to low dose cellular exposure, namely the adaptive response. This effect of low dose radiation on cells was first demonstrated by Olivieri *et al* [96] after observing that human lymphocytes growing in radioactive thymidine solution were more resistant to the effect of subsequent high doses of radiation than the control group grown in non-radioactive culture. Cellular radioresistance to subsequent doses was materialised through a reduction of chromosomal aberrations.

In vitro experimental studies have shown that the two low-dose phenomena: the bystander effect and the adaptive response basically coexist. However, their effect on cells works in opposition, as bystander effects result in excess cell kill, while the adaptive response confers resistance to subsequent doses of radiation.

According to the adaptive response model, the isoeffect per dose fraction is not a valid theory anymore, as the first dose of radiation should kill a higher percent of the tumour cell population than the subsequent doses. Furthermore, for those patients that undergo pre-treatment diagnostic examinations that employ low doses, the adaptive response might work even for the first treatment dose.

More studies are needed to explain these two effects in head and neck cancer cell lines and to determine their magnitude for the *in vivo* state.

4. Conclusions

The management of locally advanced head and neck cancers is demanding. Tumour hypoxia, accelerated repopulation during treatment and inherent radioresistance are the main culprits for the suboptimal tumour control. The Rs of radiotherapy, as described above, play an important role in treatment design, particularly when it comes to dose fractionation in radiotherapy. Questions then arise as to how fractionated the treatment should be and what other parameters should be taken into consideration in order to achieve a high therapeutic gain.

As demonstrated by clinical trials, conventionally fractionated treatments are not efficient for head and neck cancer patients. Instead, altered fractionation schedules should be employed to overcome the radiobiological challenges. Accelerated fractionation is a rather aggressive protocol that, however, is needed in response to an aggressive tumour. Treatment breaks are often scheduled in these situations to allow time for normal tissue repair. Hyperfractionated radiotherapy is a perfect way to apply the Rs of radiotherapy for rapidly proliferating tumours such as head and neck carcinomas. By giving more than one dose fraction a day, tumour repopulation during treatment is minimised and tumour reoxygenation is stimulated. Hyperfractionated schedules were shown to provide the greatest benefit among these patients.

While hypoxia and repopulation are usual characteristics of head and neck cancers, the extent of hypoxia and the degree of tumour proliferation differ from patient to patient. These pre-treatment disparities lead to different post-treatment tumour responses. Decades ago, the idea of predictive assays for tumour oxygenation, proliferation and radioresistance has been embraced with high optimism. However, due to several technical and clinical challenges, the routine implementation of such predictive assays has been hindered and other methods to characterise the metabolic properties of tumours have been designed. Advanced imaging techniques such as BOLD-MRI (Blood Oxygen Level Dependent – Magnetic Resonance Imaging) or PET (Positron Emission Tomography) can give valuable indication regarding oxygenation and proliferation. The goal to gather such information is to design individualised treatments, based on patient-specific parameters. Personalised treatment is therefore the key solution for the management of advanced head and neck cancers. This will be achieved with (figure 1):

- routine clinical implementation of *predictive assays,* which in the current era are often *PET*-based,
- *protection* of normal tissue to diminish adverse effects,
- improved *perfusion* of oxygen inside the tumour to allow for reoxygenation and better chemotherapy delivery.

These P's of head and neck cancer treatment can lead to an enhanced therapeutic ratio by increasing tumour control and decreasing normal tissue toxicity.

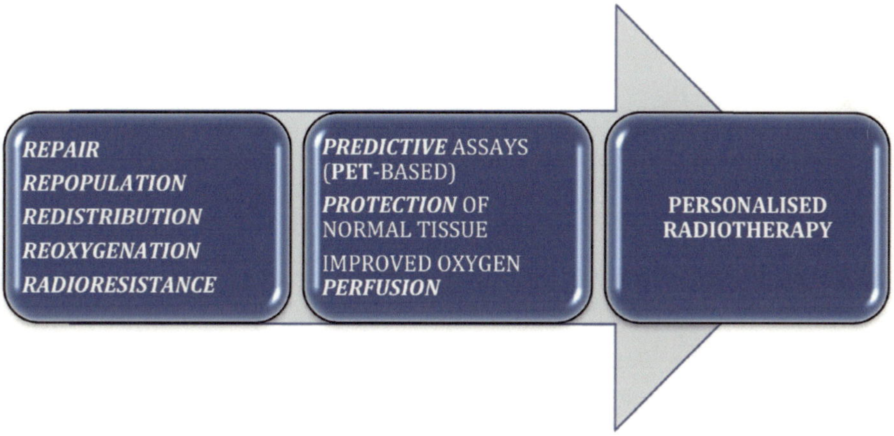

Figure 1. The Ps and Rs of head and neck cancer management towards Personalised Radiotherapy.

A more accurate patient selection for the administration of chemotherapeutical agents or altered fractionation schedules could lead to a better management of head and neck cancer with personalised treatment planning and delivery.

Acknowledgements

LGM would like to acknowledge the support offered by the Ministry of National Education (Romania), CNCS-UEFISCDI, Project no. PN-II-ID-PCE-2012-4-0067.

ITD and AD acknowledge the support offered by the Cancer Research Funds of Radiumhemmet, Stockholm (Sweden), the LiU Cancer research network at Linköping University (Sweden) and the County Council of Östergötland (Sweden).

Author details

Loredana G. Marcu[1,2], Iuliana Toma Dasu[3] and Alexandru Dasu[4]

*Address all correspondence to: loredana@marcunet.com

1 Faculty of Science, University of Oradea, Oradea, Romania

2 School of Chemistry & Physics, University of Adelaide, SA, Australia

3 Medical Radiation Physics, Stockholm University and Karolinska Institutet, Stockholm, Sweden

4 Department of Radiation Physics and Department of Medical and Health Sciences, Linköping University, Linköping, Sweden

References

[1] Withers R (1975) The four Rs of radiotherapy. Adv. Radiat. Biol. 5: 241-271.

[2] Chadwick KH, Leenhouts HP (1973) A molecular theory of cell survival. Phys. Med. Biol. 18:78-87.

[3] Douglas BG, Fowler JF (1976) The effect of multiple small doses of x rays on skin reactions in the mouse and a basic interpretation. Radiat. Res. 66:401-426.

[4] Thames HD, Jr., Withers HR, Peters LJ, Fletcher GH (1982) Changes in early and late radiation responses with altered dose fractionation: implications for dose-survival relationships. Int J Radiat Oncol Biol Phys. 8:219-226.

[5] Thames HD (1985) An 'incomplete-repair' model for survival after fractionated and continuous irradiations. Int J Radiat Biol. 47:319-339.

[6] Curtis SB (1986) Lethal and potentially lethal lesions induced by radiation--a unified repair model. Radiat. Res. 106:252-270.

[7] Lind BK, Persson LM, Edgren MR, Hedlof I, Brahme A (2003) Repairable-conditionally repairable damage model based on dual Poisson processes. Radiat Res. 160:366-375.

[8] Barendsen GW (1982) Dose fractionation, dose rate and iso-effect relationships for normal tissue responses. Int J Radiat Oncol Biol Phys. 8:1981-1997.

[9] Fowler JF (1989) The linear-quadratic formula and progress in fractionated radiotherapy. Br J Radiol. 62:679-694.

[10] Nilsson P, Thames HD, Joiner MC (1990) A generalized formulation of the 'incomplete-repair' model for cell survival and tissue response to fractionated low dose-rate irradiation. Int J Radiat Biol. 57:127-142.

[11] Thames HD, Hendry JH (1987) Fractionation in Radiotherapy. London - New York – Philadelphia, Taylor & Francis.

[12] Turesson I, Thames HD (1989) Repair capacity and kinetics of human skin during fractionated radiotherapy: erythema, desquamation, and telangiectasia after 3 and 5 year's follow-up. Radiother Oncol. 15:169-188.

[13] Denham JW, Hamilton CS, Simpson SA, O'Brien MY, Ostwald PM, Kron T, Dear KB (1995) Acute reaction parameters for human oropharyngeal mucosa. Radiother Oncol, 35:129-137.

[14] Fowler JF (1999) Is repair of DNA strand break damage from ionizing radiation second-order rather than first-order? A simpler explanation of apparently multiexponential repair. Radiat. Res. 152:124-136.

[15] Dale RG, Fowler JF, Jones B (1999) A new incomplete-repair model based on a 'reciprocal-time' pattern of sublethal damage repair. Acta Oncol. 38:919-929.

[16] Fowler JF, Welsh JS, Howard SP (2004) Loss of biological effect in prolonged fraction delivery. Int J Radiat Oncol Biol Phys. 59:242-249.

[17] Bourhis J, Overgaard J, Audry H, Ang KK, Saunders M, Bernier J, Horiot JC, Le Maitre A, Pajak TF, Poulsen MG, O'Sullivan B, Dobrowsky W, Hliniak A, Skladowski K, Hay JH, Pinto LH, Fallai C, Fu KK, Sylvester R, Pignon JP (2006) Hyperfractionated or accelerated radiotherapy in head and neck cancer: a meta-analysis. Lancet 368:843-854.

[18] Dische S, Saunders M, Barrett A, Harvey A, Gibson D, Parmar M (1997) A randomised multicentre trial of CHART versus conventional radiotherapy in head and neck cancer. Radiother Oncol. 44:123-136.

[19] Bentzen SM, Saunders MI, Dische S (1999) Repair halftimes estimated from observations of treatment-related morbidity after CHART or conventional radiotherapy in head and neck cancer. Radiother Oncol. 53:219-226.

[20] Jackson SM, Weir LM, Hay JH, Tsang VH, Durham JS (1997) A randomised trial of accelerated versus conventional radiotherapy in head and neck cancer. Radiother Oncol. 43:39-46.

[21] Wang CC, Blitzer PH, Suit HD (1985) Twice-a-day radiation therapy for cancer of the head and neck. Cancer 55:2100-2104.

[22] Horiot JC, Bontemps P, van den Bogaert W, Le FR, van den Weijngaert D, Bolla M, Bernier J, Lusinchi A, Stuschke M, Lopez-Torrecilla J, Begg AC, Pierart M, Collette L (1997) Accelerated fractionation (AF) compared to conventional fractionation (CF)

improves loco-regional control in the radiotherapy of advanced head and neck cancers: results of the EORTC 22851 randomized trial. Radiother Oncol. 44:111-121.

[23] Fu KK, Pajak TF, Trotti A, Jones CU, Spencer SA, Phillips TL, Garden AS, Ridge JA, Cooper JS, Ang KK (2000) A Radiation Therapy Oncology Group (RTOG) phase III randomized study to compare hyperfractionation and two variants of accelerated fractionation to standard fractionation radiotherapy for head and neck squamous cell carcinomas: first report of RTOG 9003. Int J Radiat Oncol Biol Phys. 48:7-16.

[24] Cummings B, Keane T, Pintilie M, Warde P, Waldron J, Payne D, Liu FF, Bissett R, McLean M, Gullane P, O'Sullivan B (2007) Five year results of a randomized trial comparing hyperfractionated to conventional radiotherapy over four weeks in locally advanced head and neck cancer. Radiother Oncol. 85:7-16.

[25] Strandquist M (1944) Studien über die kumulative Wirkung der Röntgenstrahlen bei Fractionierung. Acta Radiol. 25:1-300.

[26] Ellis F (1971) Nominal standard dose and the ret. Br J Radiol. 44:101-108.

[27] Withers HR, Taylor JM, Maciejewski B (1988) The hazard of accelerated tumor clonogen repopulation during radiotherapy. Acta Oncol. 27:131-146.

[28] Overgaard J, Hansen HS, Specht L, Overgaard M, Grau C, Andersen E, Bentzen J, Bastholt L, Hansen O, Johansen J, Andersen L, Evensen JF (2003) Five compared with six fractions per week of conventional radiotherapy of squamous-cell carcinoma of head and neck: DAHANCA 6 and 7 randomised controlled trial. Lancet 362:933-940.

[29] Skladowski K, Maciejewski B, Golen M, Tarnawski R, Slosarek K, Suwinski R, Sygula M, Wygoda A (2006) Continuous accelerated 7-days-a-week radiotherapy for head-and-neck cancer: long-term results of phase III clinical trial. Int J Radiat Oncol Biol Phys. 66:706-713.

[30] Poulsen MG, Denham JW, Peters LJ, Lamb DS, Spry NA, Hindley A, Krawitz H, Hamilton C, Keller J, Tripcony L, Walker Q (2001) A randomised trial of accelerated and conventional radiotherapy for stage III and IV squamous carcinoma of the head and neck: a Trans-Tasman Radiation Oncology Group Study. Radiother Oncol. 60:113-122.

[31] Bourhis J, Sire C, Graff P, Gregoire V, Maingon P, Calais G, Gery B, Martin L, Alfonsi M, Desprez P, Pignon T, Bardet E, Rives M, Geoffrois L, Daly-Schveitzer N, Sen S, Tuchais C, Dupuis O, Guerif S, Lapeyre M, Favrel V, Hamoir M, Lusinchi A, Temam S, Pinna A, Tao YG, Blanchard P, Auperin A (2012) Concomitant chemoradiotherapy versus acceleration of radiotherapy with or without concomitant chemotherapy in locally advanced head and neck carcinoma (GORTEC 99-02): an open-label phase 3 randomised trial. Lancet Oncol. 13:145-153.

[32] Begg AC, Steel GG (2002) Cell proliferation and the growth rate of tumours. In Basic Clinical Radiobiology. 3rd ed, ed Steel GG London, Arnold.

[33] Speke AK, Hill RP (1995) Repopulation kinetics during fractionated irradiation and the relationship to the potential doubling time, Tpot. Int J Radiat Oncol Biol Phys. 31:847-856.

[34] Begg AC, Haustermans K, Hart AA, Dische S, Saunders M, Zackrisson B, Gustaffson H, Coucke P, Paschoud N, Hoyer M, Overgaard J, Antognoni P, Richetti A, Bourhis J, Bartelink H, Horiot JC, Corvo R, Giaretti W, Awwad H, Shouman T, Jouffroy T, Maciorowski Z, Dobrowsky W, Struikmans H, Wilson GD (1999) The value of pretreatment cell kinetic parameters as predictors for radiotherapy outcome in head and neck cancer: a multicenter analysis. Radiother Oncol. 50:13-23.

[35] Hedman M, Bjork-Eriksson T, Brodin O, Toma-Dasu I (2013) Predictive value of modelled tumour control probability based on individual measurements of in vitro radiosensitivity and potential doubling time. Br J Radiol. 86:20130015.

[36] Dörr W, Hamilton CS, Boyd T, Reed B, Denham JW (2002) Radiation-induced changes in cellularity and proliferation in human oral mucosa. Int J Radiat Oncol Biol Phys. 52:911-917.

[37] Fowler JF (2007) Is there an optimum overall time for head and neck radiotherapy? A review, with new modelling. Clin Oncol (R Coll Radiol) 19:8-22.

[38] Fowler JF (2008) Optimum overall times II: Extended modelling for head and neck radiotherapy. Clin Oncol (R Coll Radiol) 20:113-126.

[39] Dörr W (2003) Modulation of repopulation processes in oral mucosa: experimental results. Int J Radiat Biol. 79:531-537.

[40] Kim JJ, Tannock IF (2005) Repopulation of cancer cells during therapy: an important cause of treatment failure. Nat Rev Cancer 5:516-525.

[41] Schmidt-Ullrich RK, Contessa JN, Dent P, Mikkelsen RB, Valerie K, Reardon DB, Bowers G, Lin PS (1999) Molecular mechanisms of radiation-induced accelerated repopulation. Radiat Oncol Investig 7:321-330.

[42] Bentzen SM, Atasoy BM, Daley FM, Dische S, Richman PI, Saunders MI, Trott KR, Wilson GD (2005) Epidermal growth factor receptor expression in pretreatment biopsies from head and neck squamous cell carcinoma as a predictive factor for a benefit from accelerated radiation therapy in a randomized controlled trial. J Clin Oncol. 23:5560-5567.

[43] Pedicini P, Nappi A, Strigari L, Jereczek-Fossa BA, Alterio D, Cremonesi M, Botta F, Vischioni B, Caivano R, Fiorentino A, Improta G, Storto G, Benassi M, Orecchia R, Salvatore M (2012) Correlation between EGFr expression and accelerated proliferation during radiotherapy of head and neck squamous cell carcinoma. Radiat Oncol. 7:143.

[44] Pedicini P, Fiorentino A, Improta G, Nappi A, Salvatore M, Storto G (2013) Estimate of the accelerated proliferation by protein tyrosine phosphatase (PTEN) over expres-

sion in postoperative radiotherapy of head and neck squamous cell carcinoma. Clin Transl Oncol. 15:919-924.

[45] Marcu L, van Doorn T, Olver I (2004) Modelling of post irradiation accelerated repopulation in squamous cell carcinoma, Physics in Medicine and Biology 49:3676-3779.

[46] Marcu L, Bezak E (2012) The influence of stem cell cycle time on accelerated repopulation during radiotherapy in head and neck cancer, Cell Proliferation 45:404-412.

[47] Nordsmark M, Bentzen SM, Rudat V, Brizel D, Lartigau E, Stadler P, Becker A, Adam M, Molls M, Dunst J, Terris DJ, Overgaard J (2005) Prognostic value of tumor oxygenation in 397 head and neck tumors after primary radiation therapy. An international multi-center study. Radiother Oncol 77:18-24.

[48] Lin A, Hahn SM (2012) Hypoxia imaging markers and applications for radiation treatment planning. Semin Nucl Med. 42:343-352.

[49] Vaupel P, Mayer A (2007) Hypoxia in cancer: significance and impact on clinical outcome. Cancer Metastasis Rev. 26:225-239.

[50] Thomlinson RH, Gray LH (1955) The histological structure of some human lung cancers and the possible implications for radiotherapy, Br J Cancer 9:539-549.

[51] Bussink J, Kaanders JH, Rijken PF, Raleigh JA, van der Kogel AJ (2000) Changes in blood perfusion and hypoxia after irradiation of a human squamous cell carcinoma xenograft tumor line. Radiat Res. 153:398-404.

[52] Dasu A, Toma-Dasu I, Karlsson M (2003) Theoretical simulation of tumour oxygenation and results from acute and chronic hypoxia. Phys Med Biol. 48:2829-2842.

[53] Dasu A, Toma-Dasu I (2008) Vascular oxygen content and the tissue oxygenation-- a theoretical analysis. Med Phys. 35:539-545.

[54] Okunieff PG, Koutcher JA, Gerweck L, McFarland E, Hitzig B, Urano M, Brady T, Neuringer L, Suit HD (1986) Tumor size dependent changes in a murine fibrosarcoma: use of in vivo 31P NMR for non-invasive evaluation of tumor metabolic status. Int J Radiat Oncol Biol Phys. 12:793-799.

[55] Rofstad EK, DeMuth P, Fenton BM, Sutherland RM (1988) 31P nuclear magnetic resonance spectroscopy studies of tumor energy metabolism and its relationship to intracapillary oxyhemoglobin saturation status and tumor hypoxia. Cancer Res. 48:5440-5446.

[56] Gerweck LE, Seneviratne T, Gerweck KK (1993) Energy status and radiobiological hypoxia at specified oxygen concentrations. Radiat Res. 135:69-74.

[57] Denekamp J, Dasu A (1999) Inducible repair and the two forms of tumour hypoxia--time for a paradigm shift. Acta Oncol. 38:903-918.

[58] Pettersen EO, Wang H (1996) Radiation-modifying effect of oxygen in synchronized cells pre-treated with acute or prolonged hypoxia. Int J Radiat Biol. 70:319-326.

[59] Zölzer F, Streffer C (2002) Increased radiosensitivity with chronic hypoxia in four human tumor cell lines. Int J Radiat Oncol Biol Phys. 54:910-20.

[60] Wouters BG, Brown JM (1997) Cells at intermediate oxygen levels can be more important than the "hypoxic fraction" in determining tumor response to fractionated radiotherapy. Radiat Res. 147:541-550.

[61] Dasu A, Toma-Dasu I, Karlsson M (2005) The effects of hypoxia on the theoretical modelling of tumour control probability. Acta Oncol. 44:563-571.

[62] Hall EJ (2000) Radiobiology for the radiologist, 5th ed., Lippincott Williams & Wilkins.

[63] Ljungkvist AS, Bussink J, Kaanders JH, Rijken PF, Begg AC, Raleigh JA, van der Kogel AJ (2005) Hypoxic cell turnover in different solid tumor lines. Int J Radiat Oncol Biol Phys. 62:1157-1168.

[64] Ljungkvist AS, Bussink J, Kaanders JH, Wiedenmann NE, Vlasman R, van der Kogel AJ (2006) Dynamics of hypoxia, proliferation and apoptosis after irradiation in a murine tumor model. Radiat Res. 165:326-336.

[65] Brizel DM, Dodge RK, Clough RW, Dewhirst MW (1999) Oxygenation of head and neck cancer: changes during radiotherapy and impact on treatment outcome. Radiother Oncol. 53:113-117.

[66] Lyng H, Tanum G, Evensen JF, Rofstad EK (1999) Changes in oxygen tension during radiotherapy of head and neck tumours. Acta Oncol. 38:1037-1042.

[67] Dietz A, Vanselow B, Rudat V, Conradt C, Weidauer H, Kallinowski F, Dollner R (2003) Prognostic impact of reoxygenation in advanced cancer of the head and neck during the initial course of chemoradiation or radiotherapy alone. Head Neck 25:50-58.

[68] Eschmann SM, Paulsen F, Bedeshem C, Machulla HJ, Hehr T, Bamberg M, Bares R (2007) Hypoxia-imaging with (18)F-Misonidazole and PET: changes of kinetics during radiotherapy of head-and-neck cancer. Radiother Oncol. 83:406-410.

[69] Zips D, Zophel K, Abolmaali N, Perrin R, Abramyuk A, Haase R, Appold S, Steinbach J, Kotzerke J, Baumann M (2012) Exploratory prospective trial of hypoxia-specific PET imaging during radiochemotherapy in patients with locally advanced head-and-neck cancer. Radiother Oncol. 105:21-28.

[70] Bittner MI, Wiedenmann N, Bucher S, Hentschel M, Mix M, Weber WA, Grosu AL (2013) Exploratory geographical analysis of hypoxic subvolumes using 18F-MISO-PET imaging in patients with head and neck cancer in the course of primary chemoradiotherapy. Radiother Oncol. 108:511-516.

[71] Thorwarth D, Eschmann SM, Paulsen F, Alber M (2007) Hypoxia dose painting by numbers: a planning study. Int J Radiat Oncol Biol Phys. 68:291-300.

[72] Toma-Dasu I, Uhrdin J, Antonovic L, Dasu A, Nuyts S, Dirix P, Haustermans K, Brahme A (2012) Dose prescription and treatment planning based on FMISO-PET hypoxia. Acta Oncol. 51:222-230.

[73] Christopoulos A, Ahn SM, Klein JD, Kim S (2011) Biology of vascular endothelial growth factor and its receptors in head and neck cancer: beyond angiogenesis. Head Neck. 33:1220-1229.

[74] Rieckmann T, Tribius S, Grob TJ, Meyer F, Busch CJ, Petersen C, Dikomey E, Kriegs M (2013) HNSCC cell lines positive for HPV and p16 possess higher cellular radiosensitivity due to an impaired DSB repair capacity. Radiother Oncol. 107:242-246.

[75] Arenz A, Ziemann F, Mayer C, Wittig A, Dreffke K, Preising S, et al (2014) Increased radiosensitivity of HPV-positive head and neck cancer cell lines due to cell cycle dysregulation and induction of apoptosis. Strahlenther Onkol 190:839-46.

[76] Begg A (2009) Molecular targeting and patient individualization. In: Basic Clinical Radiobiology (ed. Joiner M, van der Kogel A), 4th ed, Hodder Arnold, London.

[77] Bussink J, van der Kogel AJ, Kaanders JH (2008) Activation of the PI3-K/AKT pathway and implications for radioresistance mechanisms in head and neck cancer. Lancet Oncol. 9:288-296.

[78] Skinner HD, Sandulache VC, Ow TJ, Meyn RE, Yordy JS, Beadle BM, Fitzgerald AL, Giri U, Ang KK, Myers JN (2012) TP53 disruptive mutations lead to head and neck cancer treatment failure through inhibition of radiation-induced senescence. Clin Cancer Res. 18:290-300.

[79] Ang KK, Harris J, Wheeler R, Weber R, Rosenthal DI, Nguyen-Tan PF, Westra WH, Chung CH, Jordan RC, Lu C, Kim H, Axelrod R, Silverman CC, Redmond KP, Gillison ML (2010) Human papillomavirus and survival of patients with oropharyngeal cancer. N Engl J Med. 363:24-35.

[80] Willers H, Dahm-Daphi J, Powell SN (2004) Repair of radiation damage to DNA. Br J Cancer 90:1297-1301.

[81] Steel GG, McMillan TJ, Peacock JH (1989) The radiobiology of human cells and tissues. In vitro radiosensitivity. The picture has changed in the 1980s. Int J Radiat Biol. 56:525-537.

[82] Mothersill C, Seymour CB (2001) Review: radiation-induced bystander effects: past history and future perspectives. Radiat Res. 155:759–767.

[83] Mothersill C, Seymour CB (1997) Medium from irradiated human epithelial cells but not human fibroblasts reduces the clonogenic survival of unirradiated cells, Int J Rad Biol 71:421-427.

[84] Frank DK, Szymkowiak B, Josifovska-Chopra O, Nakashima T, et al (2005) Single-cell microinjection of cytochrome c can result in gap junction-mediated apoptotic cell death of bystander cells in head and neck cancer, Head Neck 27:794-800.

[85] Frank D, Frederick M, Liu T, Clayman G (1998) Bystander effect in the adenovirus-mediated Wild-Type p53 gene therapy model of human squamous cell carcinoma of the head and neck, Clin Cancer Res 4:2521-2527.

[86] Kamochi N, Nakashima M, Aoki S, Uchihashi K, Sugihara H, Toda S, Kudo S (2008) Irradiated fibroblast-induced bystander effects on invasive growth of squamous cell carcinoma under cancer-stromal cell interaction. Cancer Sci 99:2417-27.

[87] Kucerova L, Feketeova L, Matuskova M, Kozovska Z, Janega P, Babal P, Poturnajova M (2013) Local bystander effect induces dormancy in human medullary thyroid carcinoma model in vivo. Cancer Lett. 335:299-305.

[88] Cogan N, Baird DM, Phillips R, Crompton LA, Caldwell MA, Rubio MA, et al (2010) DNA damaging bystander signalling from stem cells, cancer cells and fibroblasts after Cr(VI) exposure and its dependence on telomerase. Mutat Res 683(1-2):1-8.

[89] Melo M, da Rocha AG, Vinagre J, Batista R, Peixoto J, Tavares C, et al (2014) TERT promoter mutations are a major indicator of poor outcome in differentiated thyroid carcinomas. J Clin Endocrinol Metab 99(5):E754-65.

[90] Yee Ko JM, Dai W, Wun Wong EH, Kwong D, Tong Ng W, Lee A, et al (2014) Multigene pathway-based analyses identify nasopharyngeal carcinoma risk associations for cumulative adverse effects of TERT-CLPTM1L and DNA double-strand breaks repair. Int J Cancer 135(7):1634-45.

[91] Portess DI, Bauer G, Hill MA, O'Neill P (2007) Low-dose irradiation of nontransformed cells stimulates the selective removal of precancerous cells via intercellular induction of apoptosis. Cancer Res 67(3):1246-53.

[92] Shiels MS, Gibson T, Sampson J, Albanes D, Andreotti G, Beane Freeman L, et al (2014) Cigarette smoking prior to first cancer and risk of second smoking-associated cancers among survivors of bladder, kidney, head and neck, and stage I lung cancers. J Clin Oncol pii: JCO.2014.56.8220.

[93] Dulguerov N, Dulguerov P (2013) The indication of panendoscopy in the search for synchronous and metachronous head and neck cancer. Rev Med Suisse 9(400):1770.

[94] González-García R, Naval-Gías L, Román-Romero L, Sastre-Pérez J, Rodríguez-Campo FJ (2009) Local recurrences and second primary tumors from squamous cell carcinoma of the oral cavity: a retrospective analytic study of 500 patients. Head Neck 31(9):1168-80.

[95] Yamamoto E, Shibuya H, Yoshimura R, Miura M (2002) Site specific dependency of second primary cancer in early stage head and neck squamous cell carcinoma. Cancer 94(7):2007-14.

[96] Olivieri G, Bodycote J, Wolff S (1984) Adaptive response of human lymphocytes to low concentrations of radioactive thymidine, Science 223:594–597.

Chapter 3

Immunosuppressive Microenvironment in Head and Neck Cancer

Jizhen Lin, Jinhuo Lai, Merrill Biel, Yunlu Xu and
Lieping Chen

Additional information is available at the end of the chapter

http://dx.doi.org/10.5772/60775

1. Introduction

Typically, the immune system detects and eliminates tumor cells through adaptive immunity, but that is not always the case in the local tumor microenvironment. In cancer patients, local tumor cells progress persistently—even though the bloodstream is full of tumor-specific cytotoxic T lymphocytes (CTLs), which are primed with tumor antigens in the lymph nodes and are able to kill tumor cells. In about 70% of patients with human papillomavirus (HPV)-associated head and neck squamous cell carcinoma (HNSCC), CTLs enter into the tumor tissue and become tumor-infiltrating lymphocytes (TILs). But those TILs fail to kill tumor cells in the local tumor microenvironment [1-3]. Instead, they become anergic, exhausted, or apoptotic when they are surrounded by tumor cells, especially when the tumor cells are positive for a cell surface marker called programmed death ligand 1 (PD-L1). PD-L1 is also known as B7-H1 or CD274 [4-8].

In general, about 20% of cancer patients have tumor cells positive for PD-L1. Moreover, about 20% of patients with HNSCC [9], as well as 80% to 90% of patients with orolaryngeal cancer [2, 3], are infected by HPV. In patients with HPV-associated HNSCC, PD-L1 positivity is as high as 70% [1]. PD-L1 expression in tumor cells has been shown to make them aggressive, with a poor clinical outcome. Patients with renal cell carcinoma with high PD-L1 expression are 4 to 5 times more likely to die of their disease [7]. However, the clinical outcome may be better for patients with HPV-associated HNSCC; in such patients, whether PD-L1 positivity indicates a poor or a better clinical outcome depends on tumor types [10-12].

TILs express CD3, CD8, and programmed death 1 (PD-1) surface marker proteins and are surrounded by tumor cells. In that local tumor microenvironment, PD-1 on the TIL side is inevitably contacted by PD-L1 on the tumor cell surface and activated by PD-L1. The activation of PD-1 on TILs inactivates their function. Thus, TILs are incapable of killing tumor cells in the tumor tissue. Immune negative regulatory pathways, exemplified by the PD-L1/PD-1 pathway, probably act in concert to counteract effective immune responses of TILs in the local tumor microenvironment [6].In such a context, the function of TILs is reshaped and manipulated by the tumor microenvironment, so that they fail to kill tumor cells.

Tumor cells employ several strategies to evade an immune response. An immunosuppressive network is known to exist, involving multiple immunosuppressive pathways plus regulatory cell populations, all of which can act as "checkpoints" to successfully restrict immune cell activation. The PD-L1/PD-1 pathway is the representative pathway for suppressing immune responses in tumors [13]. In certain cancer patients, this pathway deeply affects and shapes cell-based immunity and thus can serve as an immunotherapeutic target [14]. In addition, regulatory T cells (Treg), natural killer (NK) T cells, and myeloid-derived suppressor cells (MDSCs) are involved in manipulating immune responses, thereby promoting the development and growth of tumor cells. Naturally occurring immunosurveillance occurs when T-cell receptors (TCRs) interact with the peptide-major histocompatibility complex (MHC) complex; yet immunotolerance may occur when PD-L1 activates PD-1 on TILs.

PD-L1 is frequently induced by chronic infections of oncogenic viruses, such as HPV and hepatitis B virus (HBV) [15].Chronic inflammation can promote the tumorigenesis of HNSCC in all phases of malignant stages, including susceptibility, initiation, progression, dissemination, morbidity, and mortality of tumor cells [16, 17]. Conversely, the normal microenvironment has antitumorigenic forces that must be overcome by tumor cells. The typical molecule that can overcome the normal microenvironment's antitumorigenic forces is PD-L1. Accumulating evidence demonstrates that the adverse tumor microenvironment facilitates immune escape of tumor cells through active manipulation of PD-L1. The interaction between PD-L1 and PD-1 inactivates T cells, making them powerless [18].

2. Inflammatory mediators and cytokines

Generally, HNSCC is rich in inflammatory cytokines and mediators in the tumor tissue [19, 20], especially when associated with HPV infection [21]. HNSCC is characterized by profound chronic inflammation [20, 22, 23]. It is highly regulated by interferon gamma (IFN-γ), tumor necrosis factor alpha (TNF-α), and relevant regulatory transcription factors. Those factors include the inhibitor of differentiation family members, ID1 and ID3 [24], as well as immune and inflammation relevant transcription factors such as nuclear factor kappa B (NF-κB) [19, 25, 26].

ID1 is an oncoprotein that dictates the proliferation of squamous cells. An immediate-early gene, it responds to mitogenic signals, infectious agents, and bone morphorgenetic proteins (BMPs) [27]. It is an important transcription factor critical for the production of IFN-γ and TNF-α [28].

ID3 is a critical transcription factor involved in the proliferation of B cells and in antibody isotype switching [29]. Both ID1 and ID3 are involved in the adaptive immune response in HNSCC via the regulation of IFN-γ and TNF-α and via the proliferation of B cells and antibody isotype switching.

NF-κB is a well-known transcription factor activated by infection, either bacterial or viral. Clinical studies indicate that NF-κB plays an important role in the carcinogenesis of HNSCC, in conjunction with ID1 [24, 28, 30]. As shown in our recent studies, ID1 and NF-κB subunit p65 together transduce immortalized keratinocytes into malignant keratinocytes, both in vitro and in vivo [31]. In HNSCC specimens, the major inflammatory cytokines in tumor tissues include interleukin-8 (IL-8), TNF-α, and IFN-γ [19, 24]. HPV-associated HNSCC generally induces a robust immune response and has emerged as a distinct entity, with a different profile of risk factors and with a more favorable response to therapy than HPV-negative HNSCC. More than 50% of patients with HPV-associated HNSCC are infected by HPV type 16 [10-12]. The percentage is similar in patients with HPV-associated cervical carcinoma [32, 33].

Chronic inflammation is involved in tumor development and growth, in both nonimmune and immune ways, via the following mechanisms: (1) the production of reactive oxygen species, such as peroxynitrites, which promote DNA mutation; (2) the production of proangiogenic factors, such as vascular endothelial growth factor (VEGF), which promotes tumor neovascularization; (3) the production of matrix metalloproteases (MMPs), such as MMP9, which facilitate invasion and metastasis; and (4) the perturbation of myelopoiesis and hemopoiesis, thereby causing a deficiency in antigen-presenting cells, as well as dysfunctional cell-based antitumor immunity [34].

One result is the unleashing of MDSCs to dispose of dendritic cells. MDSCs are immature myeloid cells that inhibit both innate and adaptive immunity, thus subverting immunosurveillance. They are thought to be a disturbed differentiation of dendritic cells by inflammatory mediators, such as VEGF, IL-6, cyclooxygenase-2 (COX-2), and prostaglandin E_2 (PGE_2) [20]. MDSCs are present in patients with HNSCC [35, 36]—especially those with oropharyngeal cancer, [37] 80% to 90% of whom are infected by HPV. Inflammatory cytokines and mediators (e.g., IL-6, VEGF, COX-2, PGE_2,) induce the formation of MDSCs and cause immunosuppression in most cancer patients; MDSCs are an impediment to all immunotherapies that require an active immune response by the host. Blockade of PD-L1 improves T-cell activation mediated by myeloid dendritic cells, in turn downregulating T-cell IL-10 and upregulating IL-2 and IFN-γ [38].

Thus, blockade of PD-L1 is indirectly relevant to counteracting the inhibition of Treg cells. A subset of CD4+ regulatory T lymphocytes, Treg cells inhibit effector T lymphocytes. Tumor cells and microenvironmental macrophages produce chemokines to attract Treg cells into the tumor tissue [39]. Even though Treg cells inhibit immune responses, they have no value, according to many studies, in predicting the prognosis of patients with HNSCC. Nonetheless, the $CD8^+$/$FoxP3^+$ (effector:regulatory) ratio, the $CD8^+$/$CD4^+$ (effector:helper) ratio, and the Treg cell subset ($CD45RA^-FoxP3^+$) may be useful in predicting the prognosis [40-42]. PD-L1 costimulates the secretion of IL-10, which promotes the function of Treg cells [4].

2.1. ID1-IFNγ/TNFα-PD-L1 signaling

BMPs induce the expression of ID1 [43, 44]. ID1 regulates the expression of INF-γ and TNF-α in T cells [28]. IFN-γ and TNF-α are mainly produced by activated T cells and NK cells [45] responsible for macrophage activation and differentiation [46]. IFN-γ induces transcription of several proinflammatory genes, such as inducible NO synthase (iNOS), COX-2 [47], and IL-1β, as well as MHC proteins [46]. In mouse macrophages, IFN-γ regulates TNF-α expression [45]. ID1 is critical for recruiting γδ T cells into the skin tissue via CXC chemokine receptor type 4 (CXCR4), a receptor specific for stromal derived factor 1 (SDF-1). Involved in the "settling down" of tumor cells in a new organ or tissue, SDF-1 is thus implicated in the metastasis of tumor cells. *ID1*$^{-/-}$ mice are *more* susceptible to skin tumorigenesis (as compared with their wild-type counterparts) because they lack CXCR4 in their blood vessels [48] and have far fewer γδ T cells entering into their skin tissue via CXCR4.

Moreover, ID1 and ID3 proteins are required for tumor angiogenesis [49] via VEGF [50, 51]. The activation of the TGF-β1 signaling pathway downregulates ID1 expression [52], whereas the activation of the BMP pathway upregulates it [43, 44]—although both pathways act through the SMAD proteins. The effect of inflammation on PD-L1 in the tumor cells is summarized in Fig. 1.

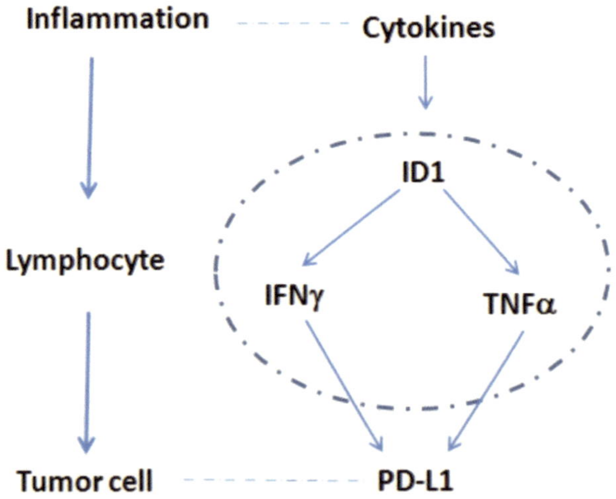

Figure 1. ID1 drives the expression of PD-L1 on tumor cells. Chronic inflammation induces cytokine expression, which, in turn, triggers the early responding gene expression of ID1. ID1 then induces IFNγ and TNFα expression in lymphocytes (T cells and NK cells), eventually inducing PD-L1 expression in the tumor cells.

3. Immunosuppressive microenvironment

At the molecular level, many inhibitory factors are involved in the tumor microenvironment. In HNSCC, PD-L1 and PD-1 interact with TILs and tumor cells [1, 13], constituting a negative signaling pathway for immune responses. The TGF-β signaling pathway inhibits the production of IL-2 and thus suppresses the proliferation of T and B cells, forming another signaling pathway for immunosuppression in HNSCC. The enzyme CD73 metabolizes adenosine triphosphate (ATP) into adenosine monophosphate (AMP), which inhibits immune responses in HNSCC. In addition, galectin-1, indoleamine 2,3-dioxygenase, and arginase might play specific roles in the carcinogenesis of HNSCC by suppressing local immunity.

Stratified by the presence or absence of PD-L1 expression and of TILs, patients with HNSCC can be divided into these 4 subsets:

1. $TILs^{+}/PD\text{-}L1^{+}$
2. $TILs^{+}/PD\text{-}L1^{-}$
3. $TILs^{-}/PD\text{-}L1^{+}$
4. $TILs^{-}/PD\text{-}L1^{-}$

About 70% of patients with HPV-associated HNSCC are in subset (1), with about 30% in subset (2). But those percentages are reversed in patients with HPV-negative HNSCC: about 29% are in subset (1), with about 71% in subset (2) [1]. In 110 human primary and metastatic melanoma studies, the distribution of patients was as follows: 38% in subset (1), 1% in subset (2), 20% in subset (3), and 41% in subset (4) [53-55]. Clearly, immunotolerance is more common in HPV-associated HNSCC than in HPV-negative HNSCC and in other subtypes.

At the cellular level, Treg cells and MDSCs comprise the inhibitory cellular populations [41]. In patients with HNSCC, as well as with numerous other solid tumors, $CD4^{+}FoxP3^{+}/CCR4^{+}$Treg cells have been shown to be upregulated [41]. In patients with HNSCC, such upregulation may potently suppress effector T-cell responses, in both an antigen-specific and an antigen-independent fashion, constituting a negative force for innate and adaptive immune responses. Treg cells make TGF-β; active TGF-β is important in order for Treg cells to mediate immunosuppression and to help maintain peripheral tolerance [56].

4. Tumor-Infiltrating Lymphocytes (TILs)

About 70% of patients with HPV-associated HNSCC have TILs in their tumors [1]. TILs provide insight into the immunologic activity against tumor cells. The presence of TILs in the tumor tissue marks an antigen-based immune response in the host. Theoretically, this action would eliminate tumor cells in the body. But in reality, many coinhibitory signaling pathways provide feedback to TILs from the tumor side and inhibit their function. For example, the PD-L1/PD-1 pathway frequently determines and controls the function of TILs or CTLs [18, 57-59]. In most cancer patients, freshly isolated TILs are usually inactive against autologous tumor cells, although they can be activated after incubation in vitro with IL-2 [60, 61]. A high level of $CD8^{+}$ TILs is associated with a favorable outcome [40], yet a low level of Treg cells has no such influence on the prognosis.

TILs predispose patients with HNSCC to a favorable response to chemoradiotherapy [42]. TILs are specific to tumor cells and are able to recognize them through the transmembrane coreceptor CD8, which binds to peptide-loaded MHC class I molecules expressed on the surface of tumor cells; thus, tumor cells are killed via the cytotoxic action of TILs [62, 63]. However, MHC class I molecules on the tumor cell surface are frequently downregulated, so the activation of T-cell cytotoxicity is impaired in the tumor microenvironment. CD3, consisting of 4 chains (ε, γ, δ, and ζ), is a pan-T cell marker and represents a coreceptor of the TCR (Fig. 2), which delivers activation signals down to subsequent pathways and eventually activates T cells. At the same time, PD-1 is upregulated when T cells are differentiated and become activated $CD3^+CD8^+PD\text{-}1^+$ T cells; thus, PD-1 is also a typical cell marker for activated TILs.

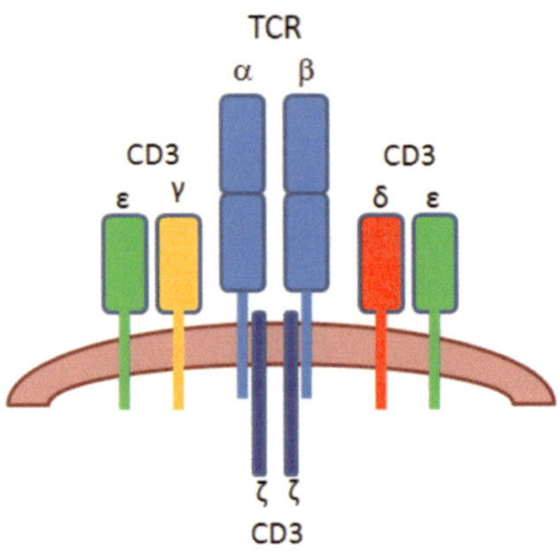

Figure 2. TCR and its coreceptor CD3 are expressed on the T-cell surface. CD3 consists of 4 chains (ε, γ, δ, and ζ), with ζ in the cytosol and ε, γ, and δ on the surface. TCR consists of α and β chains in which signals are converted into the cytosol via the CD3 ζ chain, thereby activating T cells.

Problematically, PD-1 is a surface receptor for PD-L1, which is highly expressed in patients with HNSCC, especially those infected by HPV. In that local tumor microenvironment, PD-1 receptors on the surface of TILs are inevitably surrounded by numerous PD-L1 molecules on the tumor cells and thus are activated by PD-L1. Given the inflammatory nature of HPV-associated HNSCC, a robust infiltration by $CD3^+CD8^+PD\text{-}1^+$ cytotoxic T cells in the tumor tissue is quite common. In the literature, this phenomenon is observed in different tumor types, including HNSCC as well as colorectal, breast, esophageal, renal, lung, ovarian, and anal carcinoma [40].

5. Immunotherapy

Enhancing the specific antitumor immune response is the primary goal of immunotherapy. That goal can occasionally be achieved by the nonspecific stimulation of innate immunity, for example, by activating cytokine-induced killer cells [AS MEANT?] or reinfusing TILs treated by IL-2 outside of the body. But such nonspecific measures are not effective enough to kill tumor cells in the body. In the clinical setting, a more plausible option might be to block the

http://dx.doi.org/10.5772/60775

PD-L1/PD-1 pathway, along with other possible signaling pathways (such as the CTLA-4 pathway), and to retarget T cells [14, 64, 65]. Increasing the number of tumor-specific cytolytic $CD8^+$T cells available to infiltrate into the tumor is widely believed to be a key component of effective immunotherapy; therefore, numerous approaches for enhancing the tumor antigen-specific immune responses are being actively investigated., Combined therapy with 2 antibodies (anti-PD-1 and anti-CTLA-4 monoclonal antibodies) is highly effective in patients with advanced melanoma, as compared with anti-PD-L1 or anti-PD-1 monoclonal antibody alone [66, 67]; in fact, in a recent study, combined therapy reduced tumor size in about 80% of patients [68]. Similar strategies based on that same principle might apply to the treatment of patients with HNSCC.

Because ID1 regulates both IFN-γ and TNF-α expression in lymphocytes (including NK cells, T cells, and B cells), controlling the ID1 expression levels in tumor cells and TILs is important. Activated NK cells are characterized by both IFN-γ and TNF-α expression. We and others have demonstrated, in mutant mice, that CD137(4-1BB) is a target for treatment of cancer and that application of monoclonal antibodies against the 4-1BB molecule eradicates established tumors by increasing T-cell activity [69-71]. Those earlier findings suggest that the local microenvironment of HNSCC features inhibitory forces that block the activity of tumor-specific T cells. At the 2014 American Society of Clinical Oncology (ASCO) annual meeting, results of an early-phase clinical trial of anti-PD-1 treatment (pembrolizumab, MK-3475) were presented: the best overall response rate in patients with HNSCC positive for HNSCC was only 20%.

6. Future directions

An effective strategy for reversing specific immunosuppressive mechanisms prominent in the HNSCC microenvironment is to target immune checkpoints' that modulate T-cell activity. In light of our current understanding, PD-1 and cytotoxic T-lymphocyte antigen 4 (CTLA-4) would be good choices for this purpose [72]. CTLA-4 is a negative costimulatory molecule for T cells, which are usually immature; it is the target of ipilimumab (Yervoy), an immunotherapeutic monoclonal antibody for blocking the immune proteins on the surface of TILs. Ipilimumab has been approved for the treatment of cutaneous melanoma [73]. Polymorphisms in CTLA-4 have been shown to influence the prognosis of patients with HNSCC; the implication is that CTLA-4 may be a rational target in order to block the negative regulation of TILs in HNSCC, just as in cutaneous melanoma [74, 75].

PD-1 (the negative receptor for CTLs) and its ligand, PD-L1, are both overexpressed in patients with HPV-positive HNSCC [1]. In a mouse model of HNSCC, blocking antibody to PD-1 or to PD-L1 has been shown to confer cell-based immunity [76, 77]. The safety, and evidence of antitumor efficacy, of anti-PD-1 have been demonstrated in a phase 1 clinical trial of refractory solid tumors, such as melanoma, non-small-cell lung cancer (NSCLC), and renal carcinoma [76, 77]. However, that approach has not yet been applied to HNSCC. Given the data gained from melanoma and NSCLC, a combination of both anti-CTLA-4 and anti-PD-1 monoclonal antibodies would be ideal for treating HNSCC in the future: CTLs are either inhibited by

CTLA-4 or suppressed to death by PD-1 (Fig. 3). Particularly in the subset of patients with HPV-associated HNSCC, in whom TILs are abundant, treatment with anti-PD-1 monoclonal antibody might enhance the efficacy of chemoradiotherapy.

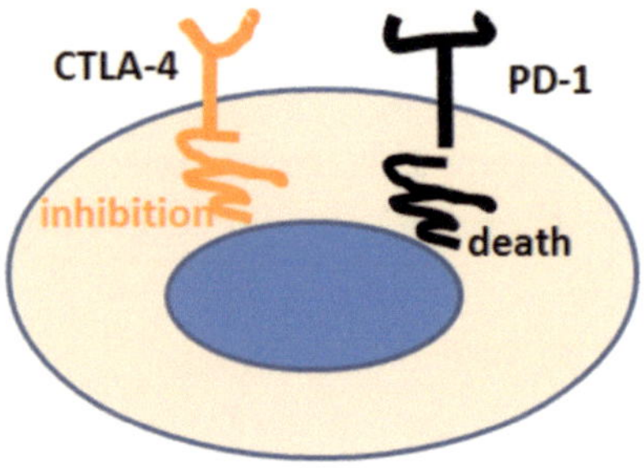

Figure 3. TILs are inhibited by CTLA-4 or suppressed to death by PD-1 in the tumor microenvironment. Blockade of both the CTLA-4 and the PD-1 signaling pathways by anti-CTLA-4 or anti-PD-1 monoclonal antibodies would be ideal for optimal activation of CTLs in the tumor tissue.

7. Conclusion

The majority of HNSCC is full of TILs in the tumor tissue. On one hand, these TILs are primed with tumor antigens and ready to fight off cancer. On the other hand, these TILs are suppressed in their functions due to the expression of PD-L1 on the surface of tumor cells. Immunotherapy is generally effective in those patients when both TILs and PD-L1 are positive. More clinical studies are needed to improve the efficacy of immunotherapy with anti-PD-1 or anti-PD-L1 monoclonal antibody.

Author details

Jizhen Lin[1,4*], Jinhuo Lai[1,4], Merrill Biel[2], Yunlu Xu[1,4] and Lieping Chen[3,4]

*Address all correspondence to: linxx004@umn.edu

1 The Departments of Otolaryngology Head and Neck Surgery, Cancer Center, University of Minnesota School of Medicine, University of Minnesota, Minneapolis, USA

2 Ear, Nose, and Throat Specialty Care of Minnesota, Minneapolis, USA

3 The Department of Immunobiology, and Yale Comprehensive Cancer Center, Yale University School of Medicine, New Haven, Connecticut, USA

4 The Department of Oncology of Union Hospital, Institute of Immunotherapy, Fujian Medical University, Fuzhou, China

References

[1] Lyford-Pike, S., et al., Evidence for a role of the PD-1:PD-L1 pathway in immune resistance of HPV-associated head and neck squamous cell carcinoma. Cancer Res, 2013. 73(6): p. 1733-41.

[2] Begum, S., et al., Tissue distribution of human papillomavirus 16 DNA integration in patients with tonsillar carcinoma. Clin Cancer Res, 2005. 11(16): p. 5694-9.

[3] Gillison, M.L., et al., Distinct risk factor profiles for human papillomavirus type 16-positive and human papillomavirus type 16-negative head and neck cancers. J Natl Cancer Inst, 2008. 100(6): p. 407-20.

[4] Dong, H., et al., B7-H1, a third member of the B7 family, co-stimulates T-cell proliferation and interleukin-10 secretion. Nat Med, 1999. 5(12): p. 1365-9.

[5] Dong, H., et al., Tumor-associated B7-H1 promotes T-cell apoptosis: a potential mechanism of immune evasion. Nat Med, 2002. 8(8): p. 793-800.

[6] Zou, W. and L. Chen, Inhibitory B7-family molecules in the tumour microenvironment. Nat Rev Immunol, 2008. 8(6): p. 467-77.

[7] Thompson, R.H., et al., Costimulatory B7-H1 in renal cell carcinoma patients: Indicator of tumor aggressiveness and potential therapeutic target. Proc Natl Acad Sci U S A, 2004. 101(49): p. 17174-9.

[8] Azuma, T., et al., B7-H1 is a ubiquitous antiapoptotic receptor on cancer cells. Blood, 2008. 111(7): p. 3635-43.

[9] Ang, K.K., et al., Human papillomavirus and survival of patients with oropharyngeal cancer. N Engl J Med, 2010. 363(1): p. 24-35.

[10] Ramqvist, T. and T. Dalianis, Oropharyngeal cancer epidemic and human papillomavirus. Emerg Infect Dis, 2010. 16(11): p. 1671-7.

[11] Lin, W., et al., Development and immunophenotyping of squamous cell carcinoma xenografts: tools for translational immunology. Laryngoscope, 2005. 115(7): p. 1154-62.

[12] Jayaprakash, V., et al., Human papillomavirus types 16 and 18 in epithelial dysplasia of oral cavity and oropharynx: a meta-analysis, 1985-2010. Oral Oncol, 2011. 47(11): p. 1048-54.

[13] Zandberg, D.P. and S.E. Strome, The role of the PD-L1:PD-1 pathway in squamous cell carcinoma of the head and neck. Oral Oncol, 2014. 50(7): p. 627-632.

[14] Brahmer, J.R., Harnessing the immune system for the treatment of non-small-cell lung cancer. J Clin Oncol, 2013. 31(8): p. 1021-8.

[15] Hofmeyer, K.A., H. Jeon, and X. Zang, The PD-1/PD-L1 (B7-H1) pathway in chronic infection-induced cytotoxic T lymphocyte exhaustion. J Biomed Biotechnol, 2011. 2011: p. 451694.

[16] Trinchieri, G., Cancer and inflammation: an old intuition with rapidly evolving new concepts. Annu Rev Immunol, 2012. 30: p. 677-706.

[17] Galon, J., et al., The immune score as a new possible approach for the classification of cancer. J Transl Med, 2012. 10: p. 1.

[18] Chen, L. and D.B. Flies, Molecular mechanisms of T cell co-stimulation and co-inhibition. Nat Rev Immunol, 2013. 13(4): p. 227-42.

[19] Ondrey, F.G., et al., Constitutive activation of transcription factors NF-(kappa)B, AP-1, and NF-IL6 in human head and neck squamous cell carcinoma cell lines that express pro-inflammatory and pro-angiogenic cytokines. Mol Carcinog, 1999. 26(2): p. 119-29.

[20] Ostrand-Rosenberg, S. and P. Sinha, Myeloid-derived suppressor cells: linking inflammation and cancer. J Immunol, 2009. 182(8): p. 4499-506.

[21] Westra, W.H., The changing face of head and neck cancer in the 21st century: the impact of HPV on the epidemiology and pathology of oral cancer. Head Neck Pathol, 2009. 3(1): p. 78-81.

[22] Srivastava, M.K., et al., Myeloid-derived suppressor cells inhibit T-cell activation by depleting cystine and cysteine. Cancer Res, 2010. 70(1): p. 68-77.

[23] Hanson, E.M., et al., Myeloid-derived suppressor cells down-regulate L-selectin expression on CD4+ and CD8+ T cells. J Immunol, 2009. 183(2): p. 937-44.

[24] Lin, J., et al., Id1 regulates the survival of HNSCC via the NF-kB/survivin and PI3K/Akt signaling pathways. Clin Cancer Res, 2010. 16: p. 77-87.

[25] Duffey, D.C., et al., Expression of a dominant-negative mutant inhibitor-kappaBalpha of nuclear factor-kappaB in human head and neck squamous cell carcinoma inhibits survival, proinflammatory cytokine expression, and tumor growth in vivo. Cancer Res, 1999. 59: p. 3468-74.

[26] Rhodus, N.L., et al., NF-kappaB dependent cytokine levels in saliva of patients with oral preneoplastic lesions and oral squamous cell carcinoma. Cancer Detect Prev, 2005. 29(1): p. 42-5.

[27] Korchynskyi, O. and P. ten Dijke, Identification and functional characterization of distinct critically important bone morphogenetic protein-specific response elements in the Id1 promoter. J Biol Chem, 2002. 277(7): p. 4883-91.

[28] Yang, Y., H.C. Liou, and X.H. Sun, Id1 potentiates NF-kappaB activation upon T cell receptor signaling. J Biol Chem, 2006. 281(46): p. 34989-96.

[29] Pan, L., et al., Impaired immune responses and B-cell proliferation in mice lacking the Id3 gene. Mol Cell Biol, 1999. 19(9): p. 5969-80.

[30] Ling, M.T., et al., Id-1 expression promotes cell survival through activation of NF-kappaB signalling pathway in prostate cancer cells. Oncogene, 2003. 22(29): p. 4498-508.

[31] Lai, J., et al., Id1 and NF-kappaB promote the generation of CD133+ and BMI-1+ keratinocytes and the growth of xenograft tumors in mice. Int J Oncol, 2014. 44(5): p. 1481-9.

[32] Chen, L., et al., Metastatic conversion of cells by expression of human papillomavirus type 16 E6 and E7 genes. Proc Natl Acad Sci U S A, 1993. 90(14): p. 6523-7.

[33] Chen, L.P., et al., Human papillomavirus type 16 nucleoprotein E7 is a tumor rejection antigen. Proc Natl Acad Sci U S A, 1991. 88(1): p. 110-4.

[34] Gabrilovich, D., Mechanisms and functional significance of tumour-induced dendritic-cell defects. Nat Rev Immunol, 2004. 4(12): p. 941-52.

[35] Pak, A.S., et al., Mechanisms of immune suppression in patients with head and neck cancer: presence of CD34(+) cells which suppress immune functions within cancers that secrete granulocyte-macrophage colony-stimulating factor. Clin Cancer Res, 1995. 1(1): p. 95-103.

[36] Young, M.R., et al., Chemoattraction of femoral CD34+ progenitor cells by tumor-derived vascular endothelial cell growth factor. Clin Exp Metastasis, 1999. 17(10): p. 881-8.

[37] Brandau, S., et al., Myeloid-derived suppressor cells in the peripheral blood of cancer patients contain a subset of immature neutrophils with impaired migratory properties. J Leukoc Biol, 2011. 89(2): p. 311-7.

[38] Curiel, T.J., et al., Blockade of B7-H1 improves myeloid dendritic cell-mediated antitumor immunity. Nat Med, 2003. 9(5): p. 562-7.

[39] Curiel, T.J., et al., Specific recruitment of regulatory T cells in ovarian carcinoma fosters immune privilege and predicts reduced survival. Nat Med, 2004. 10(9): p. 942-9.

[40] Gooden, M.J., et al., The prognostic influence of tumour-infiltrating lymphocytes in cancer: a systematic review with meta-analysis. Br J Cancer, 2011. 105(1): p. 93-103.

[41] Sun, W., et al., CD45RA-Foxp3high but not CD45RA+Foxp3low suppressive T regulatory cells increased in the peripheral circulation of patients with head and neck squamous cell carcinoma and correlated with tumor progression. J Exp Clin Cancer Res, 2014. 33(1): p. 35.

[42] Balermpas, P., et al., Tumor-infiltrating lymphocytes favor the response to chemoradiotherapy of head and neck cancer. Oncoimmunology, 2014. 3(1): p. e27403.

[43] Ogata, T., et al., Bone morphogenetic protein 2 transiently enhances expression of a gene, Id (inhibitor of differentiation), encoding a helix-loop-helix molecule in osteoblast-like cells. Proc Natl Acad Sci U S A, 1993. 90(19): p. 9219-22.

[44] Hollnagel, A., et al., Id genes are direct targets of bone morphogenetic protein induction in embryonic stem cells. J Biol Chem, 1999. 274(28): p. 19838-45.

[45] Vila-del Sol, V., C. Punzon, and M. Fresno, IFN-gamma-induced TNF-alpha expression is regulated by interferon regulatory factors 1 and 8 in mouse macrophages. J Immunol, 2008. 181(7): p. 4461-70.

[46] Boehm, U., et al., Cellular responses to interferon-gamma. Annu Rev Immunol, 1997. 15: p. 749-95.

[47] Blanco, J.C., et al., Interferon regulatory factor (IRF)-1 and IRF-2 regulate interferon gamma-dependent cyclooxygenase 2 expression. J Exp Med, 2000. 191(12): p. 2131-44.

[48] Sikder, H., et al., Disruption of Id1 reveals major differences in angiogenesis between transplanted and autochthonous tumors. Cancer Cell, 2003. 4(4): p. 291-9.

[49] Lyden, D., et al., Id1 and Id3 are required for neurogenesis, angiogenesis and vascularization of tumour xenografts. Nature, 1999. 401: p. 670-7.

[50] Ling, M.T., et al., Overexpression of Id-1 in prostate cancer cells promotes angiogenesis through the activation of vascular endothelial growth factor (VEGF) Carcinogenesis, 2005. 26: p. 1668-1676.

[51] Fukudome, S., et al., Regulation of the angiogenesis of acquired middle ear cholesteatomas by inhibitor of DNA binding transcription factor. JAMA Otolaryngol Head Neck Surg, 2013. 139(3): p. 273-8.

[52] Ling, M.T., et al., Down-regulation of Id-1 expression is associated with TGF beta 1-induced growth arrest in prostate epithelial cells. Biochim Biophys Acta, 2002. 1570(3): p. 145-52.

[53] Taube, J.M., et al., Colocalization of inflammatory response with B7-h1 expression in human melanocytic lesions supports an adaptive resistance mechanism of immune escape. Sci Transl Med, 2012. 4(127): p. 127ra37.

[54] Sznol, M. and L. Chen, Antagonist antibodies to PD-1 and B7-H1 (PD-L1) in the treatment of advanced human cancer--response. Clin Cancer Res, 2013. 19(19): p. 5542.

[55] Sznol, M. and L. Chen, Antagonist antibodies to PD-1 and B7-H1 (PD-L1) in the treatment of advanced human cancer. Clin Cancer Res, 2013. 19(5): p. 1021-34.

[56] Roberts, A.B. and M.B. Sporn, Transforming growth factor beta. Adv Cancer Res, 1988. 51: p. 107-45.

[57] Zhang, X., et al., Structural and functional analysis of the costimulatory receptor programmed death-1. Immunity, 2004. 20(3): p. 337-47.

[58] Dong, H., et al., B7-H1 determines accumulation and deletion of intrahepatic CD8(+) T lymphocytes. Immunity, 2004. 20(3): p. 327-36.

[59] Zhu, Y., S. Yao, and L. Chen, Cell surface signaling molecules in the control of immune responses: a tide model. Immunity, 2011. 34(4): p. 466-78.

[60] Rosenberg, S.A., The development of new immunotherapies for the treatment of cancer using interleukin-2. A review. Ann Surg, 1988. 208(2): p. 121-35.

[61] Chen, L., Immunological ignorance of silent antigens as an explanation of tumor evasion. Immunol Today, 1998. 19(1): p. 27-30.

[62] Bhardwaj, N., Harnessing the immune system to treat cancer. J Clin Invest, 2007. 117(5): p. 1130-6.

[63] Lesterhuis, W.J., J.B. Haanen, and C.J. Punt, Cancer immunotherapy--revisited. Nat Rev Drug Discov, 2011. 10(8): p. 591-600.

[64] Bernatchez, C., L.G. Radvanyi, and P. Hwu, Advances in the treatment of metastatic melanoma: adoptive T-cell therapy. Semin Oncol, 2012. 39(2): p. 215-26.

[65] Restifo, N.P., M.E. Dudley, and S.A. Rosenberg, Adoptive immunotherapy for cancer: harnessing the T cell response. Nat Rev Immunol, 2012. 12(4): p. 269-81.

[66] Brahmer, J.R., et al., Safety and activity of anti-PD-L1 antibody in patients with advanced cancer. N Engl J Med, 2012. 366(26): p. 2455-65.

[67] Topalian, S.L., et al., Safety, activity, and immune correlates of anti-PD-1 antibody in cancer. N Engl J Med, 2012. 366(26): p. 2443-54.

[68] Wolchok, J.D., et al., Nivolumab plus ipilimumab in advanced melanoma. N Engl J Med, 2013. 369(2): p. 122-33.

[69] Melero, I., et al., Monoclonal antibodies against the 4-1BB T-cell activation molecule eradicate established tumors. Nat Med, 1997. 3(6): p. 682-5.

[70] Lin, W., et al., Fc-dependent expression of CD137 on human NK cells: insights into "agonistic" effects of anti-CD137 monoclonal antibodies. Blood, 2008. 112(3): p. 699-707.

[71] Sabel, M.S., et al., Monoclonal antibodies directed against the T-cell activation molecule CD137 (interleukin-A or 4-1BB) block human lymphocyte-mediated suppression of tumor xenografts in severe combined immunodeficient mice. J Immunother, 2000. 23(3): p. 362-8.

[72] Weber, J., Immune checkpoint proteins: a new therapeutic paradigm for cancer--preclinical background: CTLA-4 and PD-1 blockade. Semin Oncol, 2010. 37(5): p. 430-9.

[73] Hodi, F.S., et al., Improved survival with ipilimumab in patients with metastatic melanoma. N Engl J Med, 2010. 363(8): p. 711-23.

[74] Azad, A.K., et al., Validation of genetic sequence variants as prognostic factors in early-stage head and neck squamous cell cancer survival. Clin Cancer Res, 2012. 18(1): p. 196-206.

[75] Kammerer, P.W., et al., Association of T-cell regulatory gene polymorphisms with oral squamous cell carcinoma. Oral Oncol, 2010. 46(7): p. 543-8.

[76] Malaspina, T.S., et al., Enhanced programmed death 1 (PD-1) and PD-1 ligand (PD-L1) expression in patients with actinic cheilitis and oral squamous cell carcinoma. Cancer Immunol Immunother, 2011. 60(7): p. 965-74.

[77] Tsushima, F., et al., Predominant expression of B7-H1 and its immunoregulatory roles in oral squamous cell carcinoma. Oral Oncol, 2006. 42(3): p. 268-74.

Section 2

Clinical Aspects

Chapter 4

Contemporary Assessment and Management of Head and Neck Cancer Surgical Margins

Camile S. Farah, Keziah John and Jennifer Wu

Additional information is available at the end of the chapter

http://dx.doi.org/10.5772/60066

1. Introduction

Head and neck cancer (HNC) is the sixth most common cancer worldwide,[1] which includes cancers of the aerodigestive tract, including lip, oral cavity, nasal cavity, paranasal sinuses, pharynx, larynx, oropharynx, hypopharynx, salivary glands, and local lymph nodes.[2] More than 90% of these are head and neck squamous cell carcinomas (HNSCC), arising from the mucosal lining in these regions.[3, 4]

Although oral squamous cell carcinomas (OSCC) can arise de novo from clinically normal appearing mucosa,[5, 6] they are typically preceded by clinically apparent changes in the tissue, termed oral potentially malignant lesions (OPML) and include leukoplakia, erythroplakia, oral submucous fibrosis, oral lichen planus and actinic keratosis.[7-9] Oral epithelial dysplasia (OED) is a histopathologic diagnosis that describes this tissue transformation and is characterised by cellular and morphological changes similar to those in OSCC but are limited to epithelial cells and remain non-invasive, hence termed premalignant or potentially malignant.[10] The histological grading system developed by the World Health Organisation is used widely to describe the degree of OED in oral mucosa – mild, moderate and severe dysplasia, and carcinoma in situ.[10] The histopathological diagnosis of OED, and its severity as interpreted by pathologists, is used as a predictor of a lesion's risk of malignant transformation, and also the type of intervention required – surgical treatment or watchful waiting.[11] However, a recent study found that this system was not useful for predicting patient outcomes or determining management strategies and recommended definitive treatment of all OED until a more reliable progression/transformation system is developed.[10] In addition, the presence of a non-homogeneous mucosal lesion has been shown to be a significant independent clinical indicator of underlying OED.[8]

Despite the reported transformation rate of 31.4% of OPMLs to OSCC,[12] clinical and histological characteristics have limited potential as predictors of transformation and do not aid in early diagnosis of HNSCC.[5, 13] It has been shown that as many as 50% of HNSCCs may arise from apparently clinically normal mucosa, thus posing an inherent diagnostic challenge.[5, 6] Although it is established that OPML and OED are statistically more likely to progress to cancer, the actual underlying mechanisms are poorly understood, and it is not inevitable that a dysplastic lesion will progress to cancer.[5, 6] Thus upon clinical diagnosis of HNSCC, the disease staging is often advanced with worsened prognosis.[5, 11]

The diagnostic process for OPML, OED or suspected HNSCC involves visual and tactile inspection using white light and other adjunctive visual aids, histopathological assessment of a biopsy sample, and one or more diagnostic imaging methods by radiography or molecular methods (positron emission tomography (PET), computerised tomography (CT), magnetic resonance imaging (MRI)).[14] All these approaches are necessary to aid in accurate tumour staging which directs therapeutic planning, and have to overcome significant challenges including delineation of tumour volume and accurate location, cervical lymph node involvement, distant metastasis, and presence of second primary tumours.[15] The main treatment modality for HNSCC, determined at the stage of diagnosis, continues to be surgical resection in combination with chemoradiotherapy depending on anatomical location.[16] Stratified treatment approaches exist based on HPV status. Newer treatment modalities involve drug/molecular targets used in conjunction with radionuclide tracers leading to personalised medicine.[14, 17] However, despite advanced techniques for early detection and management of HNSCC, the 5-year survival rate of smoking associated HNSCC is still 30-50%, with survivors experiencing poor quality of life.[4, 18] Overall, patients with advanced disease continue to have a poor prognosis and high locoregional and distant recurrences,[19] supporting the need for hybrid technologies both pre-, post-, and during surgery to attain maximum information in minimum time.

2. Surgical margin assessment

The aim of cancer surgery is to remove as much diseased tissue and retain as much healthy tissue as possible.[20] The key issue with surgical management of OSCC is predicting the risk of locoregional relapse, reported to occur in up to 20% of cases, accounting for ongoing modest survival rates.[21-24] One key predictor of locoregional relapse is the presence of carcinoma in or close to the surgical margins of the primary tumour, which is currently not reliably possible despite surgeon's conventional gross assessment (limited to white light tissue reflectance assessing colour and texture) and thorough histopathological examination, as relapse can occur in cases with clear margins.[19, 20, 24] Histopathological examination reports margins as clean/clear (>5 mm between carcinoma and margin), involved (carcinoma exists within 1 mm of the margin), or close (carcinoma exists between 1 to 5 mm from the margin).[24-26] Even though this method has a reported accuracy ratio of >95%, around 30% of patients with histologically negative margins undergo treatment failure raising concerns about its sensitivity.[19, 27-30] In addition, intraoperative histopathological assessment relies on the quality of samples and degree of sampling, extends the time of operation and yields incomplete results.[20]

While in some cases histopathological examination shows tumour cells in the surgical margins thus implying that residual tumour cells could still exist in patients, most patients with local relapse have histologically clear surgical margins.[24] In these cases, relapse may be due to minimal residual disease (MRD) or field cancerisation.[24] In the case of MRD, small clusters of histopathologically undetectable tumour cells proliferate leading to local recurrence.[24] The field cancerisation model describes a field of premalignant epithelium, which may be rather expansive due to the process of lateral cancerisation, containing preneoplastic cells from which the primary carcinoma may have developed, and second primary tumours (SPT) can develop, following additional genetic hits.[24, 31] Differentiation between SPT and local recurrence due to MRD must be made where possible in order to determine appropriate therapeutic measures – while the latter may be treated with post-surgical radiotherapy or resection, treatment of the former is more complicated.[24] Surgery is not feasible due to the large extent of disease and radiotherapy may even be contraindicated as it could aid in the progression of preneoplastic cells into neoplasia, and thus more intensive surveillance during follow-up may be the best option.[24]

Most studies demonstrate an association between involved or close margins and a worse prognosis,[21, 32] with involved margins resulting in shorter disease-free survival,[21, 23, 32] and shorter overall survival.[33] The presence of close margins has prognostic significance, with a recent study finding margins at a cut-off of ≤1.6mm from the tumour to be prognostic of shorter disease-free survival and shorter overall survival.[32] However, molecular changes indicating early tumour development have been demonstrated in surgical margins of tumours from the larynx, pharynx, and oral cavity considered histologically 'normal'.[23, 34, 35] The rate of local recurrence (and thus failure of treatment) even in margins diagnosed as tumour-free is quoted in studies to be anywhere from 6.9-22%.[36]

It has been hypothesized that the majority of genetic alterations may occur during the early cancer progression process and can precede the observation of certain cytological changes.[37] It is thus believed that if given a reliable set of molecular or genetic biomarkers of epithelial transition/progression to malignancy, the subsequent removal of the altered tissue may prevent the future development of malignancy at that site.[38, 39] Such molecular biomarkers may also be used to assess the margins of tumours subsequent to surgical resection,[24, 40] allowing a means of objective assessment which may detect MRD, and predict potential for local recurrence in the surrounding tissues. Furthermore, molecular studies on genetic markers have shown there is a clonal relationship between the primary tumour and premalignant epithelium adjacent to the tumour,[24] suggesting that molecular analysis of histologically negative surgical margins may be a more sensitive method for detecting malignant transformed cells.[19] Ultimately we would like to propose a shift from conventional histopathological assessment of surgical margins to molecular analysis, either through laboratory testing or imaging techniques.

3. Biomarkers in HNSCC

Since there is a need to reconsider methods of surgical margin assessment during SCC resection, margins should not only be examined macroscopically and microscopically, but also at a molecular level for dysregulated gene expression, which is also applicable in the diagnosis of OED and OPML. It is currently accepted that genetic and epigenetic changes within a clonal population of cells drives carcinogenesis by influencing oncogenes and tumour suppressor genes (TSG).[41-43]

Current modelling postulates that the development of cancer is driven by the accumulation of genetic and epigenetic changes within a clonal population of cells.[44] These genotypic alterations can affect hundreds of genes, leading to phenotypic changes in critical cellular functions such as resistance to cell death, increased proliferation, induction of angiogenesis, and the ability to invade and metastasize.[45] The mechanisms underlying these genetic and epigenetic aberrations can include genomic instability through chromosomal rearrangement, amplification, deletion, methylation, or mutation.[45]

These genetic alterations have been shown to contribute directly to cancer development and progression, and have a direct effect upon oncogenes and TSGs as well as the phenotypes they regulate.[41-43] There has been considerable investigation into the genotypic and phenotypic alterations observed in HNC,[42] and many studies have attempted to identify the genetic and molecular aberrations occurring in HNC surgical margins as a means of predicting local recurrence and relapse.

De Carvalho *et al.* examined 55 HNSCC patients undergoing operative therapy with histologically negative surgical margins and found 36.4% of these patients (20/55) showed overexpression of one of three genes they reported to being overexpressed in tumour samples – *MMP9*, *EPCAM* and *PTHLH*, with *MMP9* overexpression correlating with the risk of developing SPT.[19] Santhi *et al.* showed that both cytoplasmic and nuclear NF-κB proteins had a significant negative correlation from tumour to surgical margin to extra margin (2 cm away from the actual surgical margin), with COX-2 paralleling its expression, suggesting that these molecules are involved in tumour progression and may be used as markers in assessing MRD. [46] In a later study, they compared the expression microRNAs (miRs) in oral tumour progression and oral surgical margins.[47] They reported a decreased expression of I-miR-125a, I-miR-184, and I-miR-16 and an increased expression of I-miR-96 in the progression from normal mucosa to OED to OSCC, supported by the same pattern of expression retrogressing from extra margin samples to margin samples to tumour samples.[47]

Potential molecular markers for OSCC or OED include: protein markers (e.g. *TP53*,[35, 48-53] MMP9,[54] CDKN2A (p16),[49, 55-57*] EIF4E[58), epigenetic markers (promoter hypermethylation), {Sinha, 2009 #1258, 59-61]* microRNA expression (e.g. miR-16, miR-125a, miR-184),[47] DNA copy number changes, [50, 62-65] and loss of heterozygosity (e.g. 3p, 9p, 13q, 11q, 17p).[63, 66-68] Table 1 summarises studies that have investigated molecular markers with the potential to predict local relapse. Table 2 details the list of studies investigating the performance of molecular markers in HNSCC surgical margin analysis using a case (with relapse) and control (without local relapse) approach, with the development of local relapse being the end-point.

Study	Marker (analysis method)	Patients and Tumours	Samples studied	Results (number of positive/total)	Notes
Jin et al.[292]	TP53 mutation (PCR-SSCP)	Laryngeal carcinoma (n = 20)	Tumour-adjacent tissue histologically normal	5/20	
Cruz et al.[48]	TP53 mutation (IHC)	OSCC (n = 42)	Tumour-adjacent tissue non-malignant mucosa	7/42	
Tunca et al.[51]	TP53 mutation (PCR-SSCP and sequencing)	HNSCC (n = 15)	Surgical margin tissue	5/15	
Van der Toorn et al.[293]	TP53 mutation (IHC)	OSCC (n = 20)	Tumour-free surgical margin	11/20	
Blide et al.[49]	TP53 mutation, CDKN2A (p16), CHEK2, LAMA5 (via IHC)	OSCC (n = 16)	Tumour-free surgical margin	12/16 (TP53) 11/16 (p16) 1/16 (CHEK2) 0/16 (LAMA5)	
Shin et al.[294]	TP53 mutation (IHC)	HNSCC (n = 31)	Tumour-adjacent normal epithelium	6/31	
Van Houten et al. [94]	TP53 mutation (IHC)	HNSCC (n = 30)	Tumour-free surgical margin	19/30	Only margin samples with TP53 mutation in tumour were investigated
Nathan et al.[54]	TP53 mutation, 4E, MMP-9 (via IHC)	HNSCC (n = 52)	Tumour-free surgical margin	- 23/52 (TP53) - 27/52 (4E) - 28/52 (MMP-9)	
Tabor et al.[82]	Microsatellite (LOH)	HNSCC (n = 28)	- Tumour-adjacent non-malignant mucosa samples (n = 140) - Tumour-free surgical margins (n = 42)	- 10/28 - 7/28	
Szukala et al.[295]	Microsatellite (LOH at 13q)	Laryngeal carcinoma (n = 65)	Cancer-free surgical margin	8-20/65	
Poh et al.[68]	Microsatellite (LOH at 3p and 9p)	OSCC (n = 20)	Tumour-adjacent tissue, cancer free (n = 32)	15/32	
Breiger et al.[67]	Microsatellite at 3q26	HNSCC (n = 20)	- Biopsy 1cm from tumour (n = 20)	- 4/20 - 3/20	

Study	Marker (analysis method)	Patients and Tumours	Samples studied	Results (number of positive/total)	Notes
			- Biopsy 2cm from tumour (n = 20)		
Bremmer et al.[63]	Microsatellite (LOH at 3p, 9p, 11q and 17p), DNA ploidy, MLPA	HNSCC (n = 10)	Cancer-free surgical margin	- 10/10 - 4/10 - 10/10	Only margins with TP53 mutations were analysed
Martone et al.[55]	Promoter hypermethylation of MGMT, CDKN2A (p16), DAPK1	HNSCC (n = 11)	Cancer-free surgical margin	5/11 (MGMT) 3/11 (CDKN2A (p16)) 8/11 (DAPK1)	
Goldenberg et al. [34]	Promoter hypermethylation MGMT and CDKN2A (p16)	HNSCC (n = 6)	Surgical margins	3/6	Intraoperative margin analysis
Wong et al.[57]	Promoter-methylation CDKN2A (p16) and p15	HNSCC (n = 73)	Tumour-adjacent mucosa histologically normal (n = 29)	5/29 (CDKN2A (p16)) 18/29 (p15)	
Supic et al.[61]	Promoter hypermethylation of p16, DAPK, RASSF1A, APC, WIF1, RUNX3, E-cad, MGMT, hMLH1	OSCC (n = 47)	Tumour-adjacent mucosa histologically normal	44/47 (any marker) 27/47 (p16) 14/47 (DAPK) 17/47 (RASSF1A) 6/47 (APC) 19/47 (WIF1) 11/47 (RUNX3) 6/47 (E-cad) 7/47 (MGMT) 6/47 (hMLH1)	
Shaw et al.[296]	Promoter hypermethylation of p16, CYGB (via PMA)	OSCC (n = 20)	Deep margins histologically tumour-free	11/20 (p16) 17/20 (CYGB)	Possible contamination from adjacent tumour

Study	Marker (analysis method)	Patients and Tumours	Samples studied	Results (number of positive/total)	Notes
Roh et al.[60]	Promoter hypermethylation of p16, DCC, KIF1A, EDNRB (via qMSP)	HNSCC (n = 12)	Deep margins grossly tumour-free	8/12 (any marker)	
Kato et al.[72]	Promoter hypermethylation of p16, MGMT (via MSP)	OSCC (n = 51)	Tumour-adjacent mucosa histologically normal (n = 22)	6/22 (p16) 9/22 (MGMT)	
Barrera et al.[297]	Chromosome imbalance (Interphase-FISH)	HNSCC (n = 10)	Cell brushings of clinically normal tumour-adjacent margins	10/10	Possible contamination from adjacent tumour
Voravud et al. [298]	Chromosome imbalance (Interphase-FISH)	HNSCC (n = 20)	Epithelium adjacent to tumour, histologically normal	8/20	
Ott et al.[62]	Chromosome imbalance (Interphase-FISH)	HNSCC (n = 20)	Tumour-adjacent margins	Most cases/20 (any genomic change)	Various chromosomes targeted
Stafford et al.[64]	Chromosome imbalance (CGH)	HNSCC (n = 19)	Clinically normal tumour-adjacent mucosa	0/19	
Fabricius et al. [299]	Telomerase (DNA-PCR)	HNSCC (n = 40)	Tumour margin biopsy	13/40	
Preuss et al.[65]	DNA Ploidy	HNSCC (n = 20)	- Biopsy 1cm from tumour (n = 20) - Biopsy 2cm from tumour (n = 20)	Greater DNA irregularity at 1cm than 2cm	
De Carvalho et al. [19]	Expression of PTHLH, EPCAM, MMP-9,	HNSCC (n = 55)	Tumour-adjacent mucosa histologically normal	20/55 (any marker) 13/55 (MMP-9) 6/55 (EPCAM) 5/55 (PTHLH)	

Study	Marker (analysis method)	Patients and Tumours	Samples studied	Results (number of positive/total)	Notes
Graveland et al. [300]	LY6D (qRT-PCR)	HNSCC (n=55)	'Clean' or 'close' deep margins histologically tumour-free	12/55	
Dasgupta et al. [301]	Mitochondrial DNA (mtDNA) mutation	HNSCC (n = 50)	Histologically normal margins (n = 24)	17/24	Only margins with mtDNA mutation in tumour were assessed
Santhi et al.[47]	microRNA expression	OSCC (n = 84)	- Surgical margin tissues (histologically mild to moderate dysplastic) - Extra margin tissue (histologically normal) (n = 56)	- Increased expression (miR-125a, miR-184, miR-16) in margin vs. tumour - Decreased expression (miR-96) in margin vs. tumour	

Table 1. Molecular markers at HNSCC surgical margins with potential to predict local relapse

Study	Marker (analysis method)	Patients and margins	(Number of patients with positive molecular margins/total patients)	Sensitivity (positive margins/ number of cases)	Specificity (negative margins/ number of controls)	Significance	Notes
Brennan et al. [93]	TP53 mutation (Sanger sequencing)	HNSCC (n = 30) Evaluated (n = 25) Margins (n = 72)	13/25 (48%)	5/5 (100%)	12/20 (60%)	Yes (KM-logrank)	
Van Houten et al.[97]	TP53 mutation (Sanger sequencing)	HNSCC (n = 179) Evaluated (n = 76) Margins (4 to 5 per tumour, 3-4 superficial	50/76 (66%)	9/9 (100%)	25/62 (40%)	Yes (KM-logrank)	

Study	Marker (analysis method)	Patients and margins	(Number of patients with positive molecular margins/total patients)	Sensitivity (positive margins/ number of cases)	Specificity (negative margins/ number of controls)	Significance	Notes
		and 1 deep mucosal margin)					
Bergshoeff et al.[50]	TP53 mutation (IHC), Chromosome instability (CIN) (via Interphase-FISH)	OSCC (n = 20) Evaluated (n = 19)	8/19 (42%)	3/4 (75%) – TP53 4/4 (100%) - CIN	10/15 (67%) - TP53 11/15 (73%) - CIN	No – TP53 (Fisher-exact test) Yes - CIN (Fisher-exact test)	
Huang et al. [302]	TP53 mutation (Sanger sequencing)	OSCC (n = 58) Evaluated (n = 25)	16/25 (64%)	11/13 (85%)	7/12 (58%)	Yes (KM-logrank)	
Partridge et al. [35]	TP53 mutation (p53 phage plaque assay, immunocytochemistry, FASAY)	OSCC (n = 18) Evaluated (n = 11)	6/11 (55%)	4/5 (80%)	4/6 (67%)	Not performed	
Nathan et al. [110]	TP53 mutation (IHC), eIF4E (IHC)	Laryngeal carcinomas (n = 54)	6/54 (11%) - TP53 32/54 (59%) – EIF4	6/23 (26%) – TP53 21/25 (84%) – EIF4	31/31 (100%) – TP53 18/29 (82%) – EIF4	Yes (KM-logrank)	
Graveland et al.[52]	TP53 mutation (IHC), LOH (PCR), Ki-67 (IHC)	HNSCC (n = 35)	17/35 (49%) - LOH	11/16 (69%) – LOH (75%) – positive TP53 staining (62%) – positive TP53 with >5% total epithelium positive (62%) - LOH 9p present (88%) – LOH 9p and/or >5% TP53 staining positive	6/19 (31%) – LOH (47%) – positive TP53 staining (84%) – positive TP53 with >5% total epithelium positive (74%) - LOH 9p present (63%) – LOH 9p and/or >5% TP53 staining positive	Yes - LOH 9p and/or >5% TP53 staining positive (KM-logrank) No – Ki-67 (KM-logrank)	

Study	Marker (analysis method)	Patients and margins	(Number of patients with positive molecular margins/total patients)	Sensitivity (positive margins/ number of cases)	Specificity (negative margins/ number of controls)	Significance	Notes
Pena Murillo et al.[95]	TP53 mutation, Ly-6D (qRT-PCR)	OSCC (n = 142) Evaluable (n = 102) Carcinoma-free resection margins	51/102 (50%) – TP53 14/51 (27%) – Ly-6D	(92%) – TP53 (42%) – Ly-6D (70%) – Combined TP53 and Ly-6D	(56%) – TP53 (81%) – Ly-6D (70%) – Combined TP53 and Ly-6D	Yes – TP53 (KM-logrank) No – Ly-6D (KM-logrank)	46 cases received post-op radiotherapy Only wild-type TP53 positive margins were analysed for Ly-6D
Yi et al.[96]	TP53 mutation, Cyclin D1, eIF4E (ISH)	Laryngeal carcinoma (n = 115)	47/115 (41%) – TP53 34/115 (30%) - D1 35/115 (30%) - eIF4E	21/33 (64%) – TP53 17/33 (51%) - D1 28/33 (85%) - eIF4E	56/82 (68%) – TP53 65/82 (79%) - D1 75/82 (91%) - eIF4E	Yes (Chi-square)	
Nathan et al. [58]	eIF4E (IHC)	HNSCC (n = 65)	36/65 (55%)	20/22 (91%)	27/43 (63%)	Yes (KM-logrank)	
Ogbureke et al. [303]	Bone sialoprotein (BSP), Dentin sialophosphoprotei n (DSSP), Osteopontin (OPN), MMP-9 (via IHC)	OSCC (n = 20) Surgical margins (histologically negative) (n = 200)	10/20 (50%) – BSP 14/20 (70%) – DSPP 14/20 (70%) – OPN 16/20 (80%) MMP-9	6/9 (67%) – BSP 8/9 (89%) – DSPP 7/9 (78%) – OPN 6/9 (67%) MMP-9	4/11 (36%) – BSP 6/11 (55%) – DSPP 7/11 (64%) – OPN 10/10 (100%) MMP-9	Yes (KM-logrank)	
Reis et al. [304]	4-gene signature of MMP-1, COL4A1, P4HA2, THBS2 (via qRT-PCR)	OSCC (n = 30) Margins (n = 136)	Not reported	Not reported	Not reported	Yes (KM-logrank)	All four genes were up-regulated in margins of patients with disease recurrence compared to those without recurrence.
Monteobugnol i et al. [305]	Ki-67 expression	OSCC (n = 42)	13/42 (30%) - High Ki-67 values	2/4 (50%) - High Ki-67 values	25/38 (65%) - High Ki-67 values	Yes (KM-logrank)	

Study	Marker (analysis method)	Patients and margins	(Number of patients with positive molecular margins/total patients)	Sensitivity (positive margins/ number of cases)	Specificity (negative margins/ number of controls)	Significance	Notes
			29/42 (69%) – Low Ki-67 values	1/4 (25%) - Low Ki-67 values	9/38 (24%) - Low Ki-67 values		
Sardi et al.[86]	Microsatellite analysis (MSI and LOH)	HNSCC (n = 41)	11/25 (44%)	7/8 (88%)	13/17 (76%)	Yes (KM-logrank)	
Temam et al. [306]	Microsatellite analysis (MSI)	HNSCC (n = 76) Evaluated (n = 26) Margins (n = 113)	7/26 (27%)	5/5 (100%)	19/21 (90%)	Yes (KM-logrank)	
Handschel et al.[307]	DNA ploidy	HNSCC (n = 40)	16/40 (40%)	14/20 (70%)	18/20 (90%)	Not reported	
Zhao et al. [308]	CD44v6, BIRC5 (survivin) (via IHC)	Laryngeal carcinoma (n = 146) Evaluated (n = 112)	35/112 (31%) CD44v6 44/112 (39%) BIRC5	20/41 (49%) CD44v6 26/41 (63%) BIRC5	56/71 (79%) CD44v6 53/71 (75%) BIRC5	Yes (univariate cox-proportional hazard)	
Schaaij-Visser et al. [309]	KRT4 (cytokeratin 4), CRNN (cornulin) (via IHC)	HNSCC (n = 46)	23/46 (50%) 23/46 (50%)	17/23 (74%) 16/23 (70%)	17/23 (74%) 16/23 (70%)	Yes (KM-logrank)	
Sinha et al.[56]	Methylation of CDKN2A (p16)	OSCC (n = 30)	13/30 (43%)	5/6 (67%)	16/24 (67%)	Yes (KM-logrank)	
Tan et al.[59]	Methylation of CDKN2A (p16, CCNA1, DCC	HNSCC (n = 42) Evaluated (n = 27)	11/27 (41%)	5/5 (100%)	16/22 (73%)	Yes (KM-logrank)	

Table 2. Performance of molecular markers in HNSCC surgical margin analysis of patients with (cases) and without (controls) local relapse [adapted and modified from Braakhuis *et al.*[24]

3.1. Epigenetic events

Unlike genetic alterations, epigenetic changes are heritable and potentially reversible.[69] Epigenetic changes refer to any heritable modifications in gene expression without alterations of the DNA sequence; they occur more frequently than gene mutations and may persist for the entire cell life and even for multiple generations.[43] The transcription of each gene may change from high-level expression to complete silencing, depending on the influence of the "epimutations" which interfere with the action of activators and suppressors on specific promoters in the chromatin context.[41] Epigenetic inheritance includes DNA methylation, histone modifications and RNA-mediated silencing.

Promoter hypermethylation is a well-documented mechanism for tumour-specific alteration of suppressor gene activity in human malignancy, including head and neck cancer.[70] In normal tissues, unmethylated cytosine is found in high densities in CpG islands; areas with high concentration of cytosine and guanine that map close to a promoter region in 40% of mammalian genes.[41] This unmethylated state is associated with a high rate of transcriptional activity; vital for maintaining TSG levels. Where hypermethylation of TSG occurs (via the enzyme DNA methyltransferase), stable transcriptional silencing of tumour suppressor activity occurs.[42, 69]

Studies have shown that methylation of the p16INK4a gene is a frequent event in primary HNC, with hypermethylation occurring in 50-73% of cases.[34, 71] In an analysis of 22 OSCC cases where paired cancerous tissues and the surrounding normal mucosa were simultaneously analysed, methylation of p16 and O6-methylguanine-DNA-methyltransferase (MGMT; a gene which produces a DNA repair enzyme essential for removing adducts caused by alkylating agents) were shown in 27-40% of specimen margins considered 'normal'.[72] In a recent study on the prognostic significance of tumour-related gene hypermethylation in cancer-free surgical margins of OSCC, Supic *et al.* selected a number of genes involved in a wide range of cellular processes for analysis.[61] These included cell cycle control (*p16*), apoptosis (*DAPK* and *RASSF1A*), *Wnt* signalling (*APC, WIF1* and *RUNX3*), cell–cell adhesion (*E-cad*), and DNA repair (*MGMT* and *hMLH1*).[61] Results showed that whilst DNA hypermethylation in histologically negative surgical margins is a frequent event, hypermethylation of p16 did not have prognostic significance.[61] Sinha *et al.* found that patients with positive molecular margins for p16 hypermethylation had a 6.3-fold increased risk of having local recurrence compared to patients with negative margins.[56] However, positivity of margins did not show any significant correlation with T classification, nodal status, histological presence or status of marginal dysplasia, or any other patient or tumour parameter.[56] However, in a recent systematic review and meta-analysis of literature, Rainsbury *et al.* concluded that based on 6 studies analysed, significantly better overall survival rates was seen in p16-positive oropharyngeal squamous cell carcinoma (OPSCC) tumours.[73] Differences in methodologies and cut-off points for analysis between the studies remain a limitation for analysis, and there remains inadequate evidence at this time to determine whether or not hypermethylation of p16 can be used as a biomarker for use in determination of clear surgical resection margins or to predict the risk of local relapse.

3.2. Loss of heterozygosity

Loss of heterozygosity (LOH) may occur when one copy of a polymorphic marker with two slightly different alleles is lost or amplified (allelic gain).[45] LOH in key chromosomal loci represents one of the more promising markers; consistently being identified as a potentially independent risk predictor, supported by data from several laboratories, including studies by Sidransky, Califano, Mao, Hong, Lippman, and Lee.[12, 74-78]

Califano and Sidransky developed genetic progression models based on their studies of gene alterations in squamous cell carcinoma of the head and neck.[79, 80] They reported LOH at 9p21, 3p and 17p13 in squamous hyperplasia, as well as LOH at 13q11, 13q21 and 14q31 in dysplasia, with loss of chromosomal region 9p21 being the most common genetic alteration in HNSCC (occurring in 70-80% of dysplastic lesions of the oral mucosa).[75, 79] Consensus has emerged that LOH at 3p and 9p provides evidence of the accumulation of genetic damage in potentially malignant lesions.[40, 81, 82] This has led to a number of investigations into the predictive value of LOH at these specific chromosomal loci in malignant risk of low-grade OED.[83-85] There is a general trend for lesions with greater disturbance in cellular architecture and organization to harbor more genetic alterations at 3p and 9p, however this is not noted in all studies. [40, 74, 76, 80]

Bremmer *et al.* implemented a range of genetic assays to screen for oral pre-malignant fields in histologically 'normal' mucosa, and concluded that LOH may be a valuable screening tool to detect oral pre-malignant fields in high risk patients.[63] The utility of LOH to evaluate risk of local recurrence in surgical margins was also noted by Sardi *et al.*[86] However, a study by Szukala *et al.* found no predictive value of LOH to determine risk of local relapse in laryngeal cancer patients, with a low frequency of LOH detected in collected 'clean' margin samples.[66]

The predictive and prognostic capacity of LOH at 3p and 9p to predict risk of transition from OED to malignancy has also been recently explored. A study by Zheng *et al.* in 2012 aimed to prospectively validate their retrospective "2000 LOH progression model" proposed by Rosin *et al.*[84, 87] Using a prospective cohort of 296 subjects with a histologic diagnosis of primary mild/moderate dysplasia, the authors first validated their original model for predicting progression to severe dysplasia, carcinoma in situ, or invasive cancer.[84, 88] High-risk (3p and/or 9p LOH) lesions were found to have a 22.6-fold increased risk of progression when compared with the low-risk (3p and 9p retention) lesions; findings consistent with the previous study.[84, 87] By further refining their model with the inclusion of two further markers (4q and 17p), prospective validation of the new model was performed. It demonstrated that low-grade lesions showing retention of 9p had approximately a 5% risk of progression over 5 years to severe dysplasia or more advanced disease.[87] This finding has important implications, as it could suggest that individuals falling into this category might not require aggressive treatment or monitoring despite having a histologic diagnosis of dysplasia. Conversely, a high-progression rate (approximately 65%) for high-risk lesions was found, and would suggest that this group should be aggressively monitored for clinical progression.[87]

From this study, a number of areas for future investigation arise. It is important to evaluate the capacity of LOH to predict risk of progression within the immediate surrounding field and of secondary oral malignancy, given that a portion of HNSCC may not arise from the exact site of the visually distinguished pre-malignancy.[85, 88]

Ultimately, comparison amongst existing studies is hindered by methodological differences, adjustment for confounders, and controls. Whilst early evidence appears promising, the clinical utility of LOH in 3p and 9p as a predictive tool to screen for progression of OED at surgical resection margins still requires further long-term prospective validation and/or investigation.[45, 84]

3.3. p53 family

p53 is a TSG located on chromosome 17p13, and plays a major role in cell-cycle progression, cellular differentiation and DNA repair and apoptosis.[89, 90] Loss of p53 function impairs the regulation of cell cycle arrest and apoptosis, thus altering the ability of cells to respond to stress or damage (such as DNA damage, hypoxia, and oncogene activation).[89, 90] This can then lead to genomic instability, and the accumulation of additional genetic alterations.[91] Loss of p53 has long been implicated in early carcinogenesis, including HNSCC.[92]

Several studies have investigated the expression of p53 in HNSCC tumour resection margins.[24, 49] Three groups have used p53 mutation-specific probes to detect aberrant cells in the resection margins,[93, 94] with 100% sensitivity achieved in identifying the tumours that had a local relapse in two independent studies.[93, 94] However, the assays used had a relatively low specificity (40%),[94] and contamination of margin samples by mutated DNA derived from cells leaking from the tumour could not be excluded.[93, 94] In a recent study by Bilde *et al.*, immunohistochemistry was used to analyse surgical specimens from 16 consecutive OSCC patients with surgical margins deemed negative.[49] Histologically normal epithelium adjacent to oral carcinomas showed upregulation of both p53 and p16, but with very little overlap.[49] It was not possible to conclude whether the observed changes represented early malignant changes or simply a reaction to cellular stress.[49] In case-control comparisons using immunohistochemistry, p53 appears to have problems with respect to marker sensitivity, which may be due to the presence of mutations not resulting in protein overexpression.[83, 93, 95-97] Ultimately, there remains insufficient evidence to determine whether p53 alterations can be used as predictive markers to identify surgical margins at risk of local recurrence.

A number of studies have shown a correlation between p53 expression and early recurrence, risk for secondary recurrence, metastatic spread and more aggressive disease progression.[49, 98] Studies involving immunohistochemical staining for the p53 tumour suppressor protein, image cytometry of abnormal DNA content, and promoter methylation of the p16 tumour suppressor gene have all attempted to establish potential markers for malignant progression.[99-101] Inactivation of p53 has been associated with a reduction in post-surgical patient survival in OSCC.[102, 103] Suprabasal p53 staining was found to be correlated with increasing grades of dysplasia in a recent study by Vered *et al.*,[104] consistent with an earlier study by Bortoluzzi *et al.*[104, 105] However, Cruz *et al.*[99] did not find a correlation between grade of dysplasia and p53 expression, with Murti *et al.*[106] finding a similar level of p53 expression in biopsies of patients who did or did not progress to OSCC; thus concluding that p53 expression was not predictive of the risk of malignant transformation. p53, in combination with p16INK4a and Ki-67 alteration, has been proposed as potential markers to define high risk leukoplakia, with further validation in larger sample sizes required.[107]

Due to the many differences in study design, methodology and laboratory techniques, there are currently conflicting reports regarding the value of p53 as a biomarker for the prediction of relapse in HNSCC surgical margins. There is yet to be sufficient validated evidence on its utility in adoption for predictive assessment of dysplastic progression.

The proto-oncogene eIF4E (eukaryotic initiation factor 4E) is a eukaryotic translation initiation factor.[108] eIF4E regulates the translation of cap-dependent mRNAs, and an aberrant increase in eIF4E shifts the balance in favour of translation of transcripts that promote cell proliferation and malignancy.[96, 108] eIF4E protein is commonly elevated in HNSCCs,[109] and its overexpression in surgical margins has been found in a number of studies associated with increased risk of local recurrence.[96] In an investigation into the prognostic value of p53 and eIF4E expression in laryngeal carcinoma surgical margins, Nathan *et al.* concluded that eIF4E overexpression appeared to be a more sensitive indicator of recurrence, and suggested that it may occur as an earlier event in the tumourigenesis process.[110] A recent study by Yi *et al.* investigating the prognostic value of p53, eIF4E and cyclin D1 in laryngeal carcinoma surgical margins found similar results, finding that eIF4E overexpression positivity of margins displayed a greater sensitivity than the other two studied factors.[96] Ultimately, further studies are still required to validate and assess the clinical utility of eIF4E in the surgical margin assessment of HNSCC.

Other genes in the p53 family have also been analysed, such as p63, p73 (both structurally and functionally related to p53) and CDK inhibitor (CDKI) p21. There is again insufficient data to determine the predictive value of p63 and p73 in the progression of dysplastic HNSCC lesions, and whilst general trends have been elucidated in the literature, there is no published data that correlates p63 or p73 expression with the prediction of progression to HNSCC.[104, 111, 112] There are conflicting reports on the expression of p21 in the progression of dysplasia in HNSCC, with Choi *et al.* concluding that whilst an increasing trend in p21 expression was detected in histological progression, there was no significant correlation or progression to OSCC.[113] Future studies aimed at assessing the p53 pathway as a whole may be beneficial to further explore the mechanisms of its deregulation in dysplastic progression to HNSCC.

3.4. microRNA

There has been increasing evidence of the role of non-coding microRNAs (miRs) in the regulation of fundamental processes such as cell cycle, differentiation and apoptosis; and by extension, the impact of their dysregulation on the process of carcinogenesis.[114-117] MiRs are single-stranded endogenous, non-coding RNA transcribed from DNA, ranging between 18 and 24 nucleotides in length. They have the ability to regulate expression of other genes on a post-transcriptional level through various processes by degradation or repression of target mRNA; influencing organ development, cell differentiation, proliferation, apoptosis and stress responses.[118, 119] Recent studies have suggested that miRs may also regulate mRNA targets through less stringent mechanisms, such as binding to non-complementary regions and binding to sites located within the coding regions of transcripts.[120] Given their pivotal function as post-transcriptional regulators of gene expression, miRs affect almost every cellular process; and have been implicated in numerous disease types, including cancer.[116, 119, 121]

The role of miRs in cancer development was first established by Calin *et al.* in a study that reported a specific miR cluster (miR-15/16) was deleted and/or down-regulated in the majority of chronic lymphocytic leukemia (CLL) cases.[122] The link to cancer was further strengthened by the discovery that miR genomic positioning appeared to be non-random,[121, 122] and that a significant number of miR genes were located at fragile sites (unstable regions that have been shown to promote DNA instability in cancer cells) or genomic regions that have been linked to cancers.[123] *RAS*, *HMGA2*, and *MYC* oncogenes have been identified as let-7 targets, indicating significant tumour-suppressive importance for this family of miRs.[118, 123]

There have been many molecular studies investigating the expression and dysregulation of miRs in HNSCC.[13, 115, 116, 124-126] Using a candidate-gene approach, most have attempted to examine the role of expression and proposed targets of specific miRs in HNSCC cell lines compared to normal samples.[13, 125-128] The underlying process by which miR deregulation affects the process of transition from dysplasia to HNSCC has not yet been fully elucidated, with a main impediment being the multifactorial aetiology of HNSCC and wide heterogeneity of lesions. However, Zhang *et al.* reported that Dicer and Drosha, enzymes involved in processing miRNA, were upregulated in salivary gland pleomorphic adenomas.[129]

In HNSCC, Li *et al.* found an increased level of miR-21 expression that was negatively associated with low levels of tropomyosin 1 (TPM1) and phosphate tensin homologue (PTEN); TSGs that mediate apoptotic and cell-cycle events.[126] In the same study, miR-21 was found to facilitate anchorage-independent growth of HNSCC cells, partly through the down-regulation of TPM1.[126] This finding has been validated in further studies observing elevated miR-21 expression contribution to neoplastic phenotypes.[130, 131] It is pertinent to note that most studies to date investigating miR expression profiles in HNSCC have used cancer cell lines, and only a few have been in solid tumour samples.[13, 132] Cell lines may not reflect the miR profiles of solid tumours, as particular culture conditions and clonal selection may radically change miR expression.[128] Of the few studies which have selected specific miRs for further investigation using patient samples, Childs *et al.* showed that miR-21 was also found in neoplastic head and neck cells, and may have potential as a prognostic marker in HNC.[124]

To date, there are limited studies investigating the role of miRs in surgical margins.[47] Santhi *et al.* analysed 72 miRs reported to be differentially expressed in OSCC and detected decreased expression of miR-125a, miR-184 and miR-16 and an increased expression of miR-96 in both progressive oral mucosal samples and dysplastic surgical margin samples.[47] Langevin *et al.* found miR-137 promoter hypermethylation to be associated with poor overall survival in patients with HNSCC, but found no significant associations with surgical resection margin positivity[133]. Further studies are required to define a broader set of miR profiles within a wider range of surgical samples, and to correlate results with patient outcomes. Ultimately, there remains insufficient evidence to determine whether these alterations could be used as predictive markers to identify dysplastic progression to HNSCC.

Despite the increasing number of studies into miR expression in HNSCC, there remain few publications that have investigated the deregulation of miRs in the transition process from dysplasia to malignancy. In an investigation of miR pre-cursors in oral leukoplakia (OL), Xiao *et al.* found up-regulation of both miR-31 and its passenger strand (termed miR-31*).[134] miR-31* was negatively associated with recurrent/newly formed OL, and they hypothesized that miR-31* may play an important role during OL progression via the regulation of fibroblast growth factor 3 (FGF3).[134] This was consistent with miR expression profile findings in a prospective translational study by Lajer *et al.*, who examined global miR expression in a series of consecutive tumours and biopsies obtained from patients with OSCC and OPSCC.[128] Of the one hundred and fourteen miRs differentially expressed between OSCC and normal epithelium, the upregulation of miR-31 and downregulation of miR-375 were found to be the most significant aberrations.[128] Thus there is evidence to suggest that the upregulation of miR-31 may be an early event in the transition process from dysplasia to OSCC; however, further elucidation of its role in the progression process and its predictive value still requires further investigation.

Ultimately, whilst early results of molecular prognostic indicators such as LOH and eIF4E appear promising, the routine use of these markers for HNSCC surgical resection margins assessment is yet to be validated. Further research is required which can ideally integrate the convenience of histopathology with the objectivity of molecular panel analysis, supported by a distinct outline of clinical parameters, baseline data, and sufficiently sizable homogeneous patient populations amenable to long-term follow-up.

4. Imaging techniques

It has now been established that molecular profiling of tissue changes enable clinicians to "visualise" more of the disease, indeed diagnose altered tissue early. While macroscopic changes may be detected under white light examination and tissue/cell level changes through histopathology, molecular dysregulation may be identified using special imaging techniques. While most current methods assess tissue in the plane parallel to the lesion, methods aiding assessment in the vertical cross-section (plane perpendicular to the mucosal surface) are required to detect lesions below the mucosal surface and evaluate submucosal tumour invasion.[135]

All optical imaging techniques detect and analyse backscattered photons from mucosa.[135] Visible light (400-700 nm) is used for conventional white light inspection, however shorter wavelengths in ultraviolet (UV) and longer wavelengths in the near-infrared (NIR) regions of the light spectrum can also be used for imaging. UV and blue light are absorbed by biomolecules to produce fluorescence.[135] In order to detect targeted tumour cells, the tumour-specific signal must be significantly discriminated from the non-specific background signals, thus optimising the signal-to-background ration (SBR).[136] The visible light spectrum has relatively short penetration depths useful for imaging (<100 μm) as it is mostly absorbed by haemoglobin, and is significantly associated with a high level of nonspecific surrounding signals, resulting in a low SBR.[135, 136] NIR is less susceptible to tissue scattering and haemoglobin absorption, yielding penetration depths >1000 μm through the mucosa and a high SBR, with an optical imaging window of about 650-900 nm in which the absorption coefficient is at a minimum.[135, 136]

Optical imaging techniques using Optical Fluorescence Imaging (OFI) and Narrow Band Imaging (NBI) reflect tissue changes at the microscopic and molecular levels. Optical Coherence Tomography (OCT) and Angle-Resolved Low-Coherence Interferometry (a/LCI) non-invasively provide information in the vertical and axial planes. Raman spectroscopy is a point detection technique based on the inelastic scattering of light, also enabling molecular histopathological examination. Computed Tomography (CT) and Magnetic Resonance Imaging (MRI) are methods traditionally used to detect carcinoma and metastasis (hence staging), and assess treatment response, providing anatomical and physiological information. Positron emission tomography (PET) is a true form of molecular imaging, opening the door for drug delivery and molecular surgical guidance. Hybrid imaging methods, PET/CT and PET/MRI, offer the best of both these imaging approaches. All these methods, collectively termed "optical biopsy", are non-destructive in situ assays of mucosal histopathologic states using the spectral and spatial properties of scattered light to measure cellular and/or tissue morphology, providing an instantaneous diagnosis.[135, 137]

4.1. Optical imaging

4.1.1. Optical coherence tomography

Optical Coherence Tomography (OCT) is based on the principle of low-coherence interferometry.[135] It provides high resolution (~1-20 μm) cross-sectional images of tissue *in situ*, higher than conventional ultrasound, MRI, or CT, and comparable to conventional histology but being non-destructive, it aids real-time surgical diagnostics and an "optical biopsy" of the tissue.[138] Initial success with this modality was with retinal pathology[139] and bronchopulmonary diseases.[140] More recently, it has been deemed useful in diagnosing diseases of the oropharynx/larynx and other oral tissues.[138, 141, 142]

OCT is similar to ultrasound B-mode imaging except that OCT uses light instead of acoustic waves, measuring the echo time delay and intensity of backscattered light.[143] The system uses NIR light, split into reference and sample beams, and plots the back-reflected light from structures within the tissue against depth (up to 2-3 mm).[139, 143, 144] Since the velocity of light is extremely high, optical echoes cannot be measured directly by electronic detection, but instead uses low-coherence interferometry – the back scattered light waves interfere with the reference beam and this interference pattern is used to measure the light echoes versus the depth profile of the tissue *in vivo*.[144] OCT also uses fibre optic technology, allowing for low-profile imaging to be performed through small optical fibres attached directly to a scalpel, tissue probe, endoscope, or microscope.[144] The device is compact and portable.[144]

In healthy mucosa, the basement membrane can be easily identified at the junction of the bright lamina propria and the darker epithelium, which is lost in the presence of invasive cancer.[145] However, one study had inconsistent results, showing a deceptive change in the histological layers when compared to conventional biopsy of oral lesions (various anatomical sites).[138] The authors also noted that OCT image analysis is unique, requiring special training, and associated with a wide range of variability when interpreting its parameters (mainly epithelium thickness and status of basement membrane).[138] The authors previously aimed to generate a bank of normative and pathological OCT data from oral tissues to identify cellular structures of normal and pathological processes, thus creating a diagnostic algorithm.[146]

While OCT is useful for clinical detection of OSCC and OPML,[147] it also has potential in evaluating surgical margins for MRD in HNSCC just as it has been proven useful in cancers of other tissues such as breast,[148, 149] skin,[150, 151] vulva,[152] and prostate.[153]

4.1.2. Angle-resolved low-coherence interferometry

Angle-resolved low-coherence interferometry (a/LCI) is a light scattering technique which isolates the angle scattering distribution from cellular nuclei at various tissue depths.[137] In doing so, it is able to provide biomarkers based on morphology that are highly correlated with the presence of dysplasia.[137] It measures the angular intensity distribution of light scattered by a tissue sample, quantifying subcellular morphology as a function of depth in the tissue.[137] For each depth layer, signatures from cell nuclei are extracted by collecting and processing the angular scattering signal using a Mie theory-based light-scattering model to produce measurements of average nuclear diameter with submicron-level accuracy.[137] Studies that have investigated the use of a/LCI have confirmed that neoplastic tissue transformation is accompanied by an increase in the average cell nuclei size,[137, 154-156] thus detecting potentially malignant lesions as well as malignant lesions. The diameter of a non-dysplastic epithelial cell nucleus is typically 5-10 μm, while dysplastic nuclei can be as large as 20 μm across.[157] When this is optimized to 11.84 μm for the classification of tissue health, a/LCI yields a sensitivity of 100%, specificity of 84%, overall accuracy of 86%, positive predictive value of 34% and negative predictive value of 100% in oesophageal epithelium *in vivo*.[137, 155] This technique has been studied in animal models, *ex vivo* human studies, and more recently in *in vivo* studies, predominantly associated with cases of Barrett's Oesophagus (which is associated with an increased risk of oesophageal adenocarcinoma) and oesophageal epithelium.[137] The system is portable and the probe can be used through the accessory channel of a standard endoscope, thus providing surgical guidance.[137]

a/LCI could have a role in assessing surgical margins in HNSCC by assessing size of nuclei in the margins although currently there are no studies that have investigated this.

4.1.3. Optical fluorescence imaging

The basis of optical imaging techniques is the ability of photons to travel through tissue and interact with tissue components.[158] Fluorescence is the property of certain molecules to absorb light at a particular wavelength and to emit light of a longer wavelength after a brief interval called fluorescence lifetime.[158] Fluorescence spectroscopy, a major form of optical imaging, is a non-invasive diagnostic tool that evaluates the biochemical composition and structure of tissue autofluorescence (AF).[159] It is relatively simple, fast, accurate, and can aid in real-time cancer detection.[159] While microscopic imaging systems for intraoperative surgical margin assessment based on endogenous contrast or AF are useful, high resolution of the diseased tissue is limited to a small field of view, making it difficult to survey the entire surgical excision margin intraoperatively.[20] Extrinsic approaches are more effective, which use fluorescent dyes detected by probes.[20] The signals can also be integrated into the white light image, which enables real-time intraoperative visualisation.[20] OFI is advantageous and convenient as it can be used intraoperatively for surgical guidance in resecting malignant tissue and for pathological sampling.[160] Various devices implementing OFI, both commercially available as well as those developed by researchers, using visible light or NIR, with or without excitable dyes, have been investigated mostly in breast cancer,[160, 161] but is now being tested in HNSCC as well.[162-166]

Francisco *et al.*[159] recently showed that fluorescence spectroscopy could discriminate between oral mucosa, injury, margins, and areas of recurrence, using a homemade fluorescence spectroscopy system, at 406 nm wavelength [159] without using injectable dyes, and providing macroscopic visualisation of affected and unaffected tissue. The VELscope™ and Identafi™ are commercially available tools that use the principles of AF and tissue reflectance to discriminate between normal and abnormal tissue. These tools are described below in order to illustrate loss of AF (LAF) and diascopic fluorescence as indicators of tissue change, which provide the clinician with additional information aiding diagnosis. Miyamoto *et al.* investigated intraoperative molecular imaging (multispectral fluorescence images) to identify tumour extensions in a murine HNC model.[167] They reported 86% sensitivity and 100% specificity in the diagnostic accuracy analysis compared to histology, the gold standard. They also reported a 60-day improvement in survival rate when using molecular imaging during surgery, compared to standard surgery (37% versus 5% respectively). Thus fluorescence can be used both for diagnosis and for surgical guidance to improve patient outcomes.

The Visually Enhanced Lesion Scope (VELscope™; LED Medical Diagnostics Inc., Barnaby Canada) uses direct tissue AF to enhance oral mucosal abnormalities.[7] An external light source, in this case blue light excitation between 400-460 nm, is used to excite endogenous fluorophores (typically nicotinamide adenine dinucleotide (NADH) and flavin adenine dinucleotide (FAD)) in the oral epithelium and collagen cross-links in the underlying stroma, which absorb the extrinsic photons and emit lower energy photons which appear clinically as fluorescence.[168-173] Since each fluorophore is associated with specific excitation and emission wavelengths, changes in tissue architecture and concentrations of fluorophores (as in the case of mucosal abnormalities and neoplastic development) results in altered absorption and scattering properties of the tissue,[7] with decreased tissue AF being reported in OED and mucosal inflammation.[68, 169, 174] Under the VELscope™, normal oral mucosa appears pale green when viewed under a filter while abnormal tissue exhibits LAF and appears dark.

While the VELscope™ has assisted in the detection of OED and OSCC not visible by conventional oral examination (COE) warranting tissue biopsy and aiding in demarcating margins, [68, 175] clinicians have been advised to use the VELscope™ in conjunction with COE as LAF may also be displayed in tissues with mucosal inflammation.[176] Complete diascopic fluorescence, wherein tissues display normal fluorescence pattern with the application of pressure, can differentiate inflammatory lesions from neoplastic lesions.[176] However, the challenge of completely blanching tissues and inter-operator variation in the interpretation of partial blanching (i.e. low specificity and variable sensitivity) grades the VELscope™ as a useful clinical tool for clinically visualising abnormalities but not an accurate discriminator of the condition of the mucosa under inspection.[176] Nevertheless, a recent clinical study suggested the use of a decision making protocol incorporating the VELscope™ in routine general dental practice allows for the detection of additional oral mucosal lesions requiring specialist referral.[177]

The Identafi™ (DentalEZ, PA, USA) is a multispectral screening device which uses direct fluorescence as well as tissue reflectance to visualise intraoral tissues by incorporating three different lights which are to be used sequentially.{#1120;Bhatia, 2013 #729} The light emitting diode (LED) white light enables superior visualisation of oral tissues but cannot differentiate between OPML and other more benign abnormalities of the oral mucosa, in a manner similar to that displayed by Microlux/DL™.[7, 178] Visualisation of oral mucosa under violet light (405 nm wavelength) through the accompanying photosensitive filter glasses, assesses the AF properties of tissue, with normal mucosa exhibiting natural fluorescence and abnormal tissues displaying LAF in a similar fashion to VELscope™.[7] Despite the dubious sensitivity and specificity of this wavelength of light,[173] areas of LAF visualised were often larger than what was clinically visible which might be due to the visualisation of deeper neovascularisation and stromal changes that accompany lesion progression, thus having a potential application in the determination of surgical margins for lesion excision.[163, 164] The green-amber light (545 nm wavelength) uses the concept of reflectance spectroscopy to characterise the connective tissue vasculature.[7] The process of carcinogenesis involves angiogenesis resulting in altered vascular morphology and it has been suggested that these tissue changes can be used to determine the prognosis of oral lesions, enabling the differentiation between benign lesions and OPML.[7, 179-181] Reflectance spectroscopy uses light within the absorption spectrum of haemoglobin (400-600 nm) which would reflect the degree of angiogenesis in the tissue. A significantly reduced reflectance spectra is observed in OSCC and OPML due to greater light absorption from increased microvasculature density and oxygenated haemoglobin content in neoplastic tissue.[7]

The underlying principles have enormous potential for application. Ongoing clinical trials by our group have shown excellent lesion visibility compared to COE under incandescent light. Violet light examination provided improved lesion visibility compared to COE, and improved visualisation of lesion borders and slight increase in lesion size compared to incandescent and white light. It also has a high level of clinical utility for evaluating inflammatory pathology. However, a high level of clinical experience is required to interpret the results of AF examination as the violet light displays low sensitivity for detection of OED. The green light helps uncover subtle vascular and inflammatory patterns providing additional clinical information.

Both these technologies highlight the usefulness of detecting LAF and diascopic fluorescence, however, additional information is required to diagnose the tissue change. Molecular studies in this area aid in our understanding of the phenomena of AF, LAF and diascopic fluorescence in oral tissues, enabling more informed use of such devices and superior interpretation of changes in AF patterns. One study in oral cancer patients showed that all their tumour samples (confirmed by histopathology) had displayed LOH intraorally when a simple hand-held device, similar to the VELscope™, was used.[68] Molecular analysis in this study on margins with low-grade or no dysplasia showed a significant association between LAF samples and LOH at 3p and/or 9p, which is strongly associated with tumour recurrence after tumour removal.[68] Furthermore, this study found that LAF extended beyond the clinical visible lesion, and these areas displayed dysplasia/cancer on histology and/or genetic alterations associated with molecular risk, thus showing that the VELscope™ can distinguish between dysplasia and normal oral mucosa.[68]

4.1.4. Narrow band imaging

Narrow Band Imaging (NBI; Olympus Medical Systems Corporation, Tokyo, Japan) utilises the concept that the depth of light penetration is dependent on its wavelength to enhance mucosal surface texture and underlying vasculature.[182, 183] The spectral bandwidth of the filtered light is narrowed.[183] The system has two modes, white light and NBI.[7] In NBI mode, only blue light (400 – 430 nm) and green light (525 – 555 nm) are emitted in parallel which make blood vessels in the superficial mucosa appear brown, and the deeper larger vessels in the submucosa appear cyan.[183] Blue light (centred at 415 nm) penetrates shallowly and corresponds to the peak absorption spectrum of haemoglobin, while green light (centred at 540 nm) penetrates deeper.[183] In NBI mode, inflammatory lesions have an ill-demarcated border and can be differentiated from neoplastic lesions which appear as areas with scattered dark spots and a well-demarcated border.[184, 185] These scattered dark brown spots represent superficial blood vessels; interpapillary capillary loops (IPCL).[7] Visualisation of the vasculature, as well as the degree of dilation, meandering, tortuosity, and calibre of IPCLs all indicate the true extent of lesions and severity of pathology, thus guiding the position of biopsy and resection margins.[184, 186-188] Takano *et al.*'s[184] IPCL classification for oral mucosa is tabulated in Table 3. It has been recommended that lesions with Types III and IV IPCL patterns must always be biopsied.[189] The presence of keratinised tissue can pose a hindrance to optimal visualisation of the lesion itself.[7]

Gono *et al.*[183] used NBI in colonoscopy and upper gastrointestinal endoscopy and concluded that magnified NBI enhanced the capillary pattern and the crypt pattern on the mucosa, which are useful features for diagnosing early cancer.[190] Later, Muto *et al.* reported that carcinoma in situ at oropharyngeal and hypopharyngeal mucosal sites can be clinically recognised using magnified NBI endoscopy, confirming the usefulness of evaluating in situ angiogenesis in solid tumours in the head and neck region.[191, 192] Yoshida *et al.* validated the use of NBI with magnifying endoscopy in oesophageal lesions.[193] A case report by Katada *et al.* showed the usefulness of NBI combined with gastrointestinal endoscopy (GIE) in detecting OSCC in the floor of the mouth.[187] Further case reports and investigations also supported the use of NBI in the oropharynx,[194] nasopharynx,[195, 196] hypopharynx,[197] larynx,[198] and oesophagus.[199] Its use in determining tumour size and margins in gastrointestinal cancers of the bile duct,[200, 201] duodenal papilla,[202] stomach[203, 204] was also investigated, all with encouraging results boasting higher sensitivities and specificities than the current detection method used at the time. All these studies hailed NBI as a method with improved detection and diagnostic accuracy of cancers in areas that are difficult to examine, and critically allowing for early diagnosis, having an impact on treatment options, quality of life and patient survival.[205] It was considered that NBI would develop into a useful tool in the future pre-, intra-, and post-operative endoscopic assessment of neoplastic lesions in the upper aerodigestive tract.[206]

Type	Description/Features
I	· Normal mucosa · Regular brown dots – when loops are perpendicular to the surface of the mucosa · Waved lines – loops are parallel · Study by Yang *et al.*[189] – 17% frequency of dysplasia in these lesions, hence remain cautious and utilise clinical judgement as well
II	· Non neoplastic and inflammatory lesions, but dysplasia present most of the time · Dilated and crossing IPCL pattern
III	· Non neoplastic lesions, but dysplasia is almost definitely present · Elongated and meandering IPCL pattern
IV	· Neoplastic lesions · Large vessels IPCL pattern destruction · Presence of angiogenesis

Table 3. Summary of IPCL classification for oral mucosa by Takano et al.[184]

In a multicentre, prospective, randomised controlled trial (n = 320), Muto *et al.*[207] found that NBI detected superficial cancer more frequently than white light imaging in both the head and neck region (100% vs 8%) and the oesophagus (97% vs 55%). They reported a sensitivity and accuracy of 100% and 86.7% in the detection of superficial cancer in the head and neck region using NBI, and 97.2% and 88.9% in the oesophagus, respectively.[207] Piazza *et al.*[208] showed that 27% (26 of 96) of patients with OSCC and OPSCC had a diagnostic advantage by applying NBI and high definition television (HDTV) compared to white light and HDTV. In a later study, [209] they concluded that NBI and HDTV were of value in defining superficial tumour extension, in the detection of synchronous lesions in the pre-/intra-operative settings, and in post-treatment surveillance for early detection of persistence, recurrence, and metachronous tumours.

Fielding *et al.* combined white light and AF to the bronchoscopic and laryngoscopic assessments of head and neck cancer patients, and reported improved sensitivity but low specificity, increasing the number of unnecessary biopsies.[210] A later study combined AF and NBI for the detection of mucosal lesions during panendoscopy in head and neck cancer patients, and reported higher specificity than when using AF or white light alone, thus directly impacting on patient management.[211]

A recently published systematic review by Vu & Farah[212] on the efficacy of NBI for detection and surveillance of OPML analysed data from a prospective cohort study by Piazza *et al.*,[209] and a retrospective cohort study by Yang *et al.*;[213] both of which aimed to evaluate the efficacy of NBI endoscopy compared to WL in oral mucosal examination. Vu & Farah concluded that based on available evidence, there is a demonstrable improvement in the ability of NBI visualization to stage tumours, assess margins and detect synchronous, metachronous and recurrent lesions compared to visualization using broadband WL.[212]

A prospective study by Nguyen *et al.* utilized white light (WL), NBI and AFAF to inspect the oral cavity, larynx/hypopharynx and bronchus of 73 patients with known HNSCC, patients with SCC of unknown primary origin, and surgically treated HNSCC patients requiring panendoscopy for suspected recurrent disease.[211] The authors found a significant improvement in the detection of moderate dysplasia or worse by NBI compared to WL, and that the combined use of AF and NBI had significant implications upon mapping and guiding the surgical resection borders of three assessed oral cases.[211] This study demonstrated increased specificity with NBI for the detection of mucosal lesions.[211]

While OFI and NBI can detect tissue and molecular changes in a localised region, imaging modalities such as Computed Tomography (CT) and Magnetic Resonance Imaging (MRI) provide anatomical information, including nodal involvement and metastasis which influence staging and treatment protocol employed. Ultimately, multimodal imaging can provide additional diagnostic information than white light illumination or a single imaging modality alone.[214, 215]

Both CT and MRI involve 3D sectional imaging and have extremely high diagnostic value.[216] CT scans require ionising radiation (with shorter scan times) while MRI does not but has a longer scan time.[216] CT is currently the most commonly used modality for head and neck imaging, and can improve delineation of soft tissue pathologies with intravenously administered contrast media,[216] however MRI provides the most detailed view of soft tissues and is routinely used to visualise such tumours.[216]

4.2. Molecular imaging

Molecular imaging modalities have the potential to be indispensable in every aspect of cancer care, from early detection to staging, drug delivery, molecular surgical guidance and treatment response.[20, 217, 218] Oncological molecular imaging is defined as the non-invasive imaging of distinctive cellular and sub-cellular events in malignant cells.[20, 219] Molecular imaging probes target the production of genetically determined biomolecules by cancer cells by displaying these directly in or on individual malignant cells, in the extracellular matrix, or cells in the vicinity such as T cells, macrophages, dendritic cells, fibroblasts or endothelial cells.[158, 220, 221] For example, probes paired with positron emitters and novel target-specific anticancer drugs could be quantitatively imaged by PET, providing information on tumour biology, guiding drug development, and furthering personalized medicine.[14, 17] Diseased tissue may also be detected through this imaging modality based on hypoxia [222, 223] or pH changes.[17, 224] It is clearly useful to detect changes at the cellular and molecular level rather than rely on anatomical characteristics alone which is commonly the case at present.[20]

Tumours may be able to be characterised without biopsies or surgery, and allow for accurate staging, re-staging and drug response monitoring, paving the way towards true personalised medicine.[20] Molecular imaging modalities may also be used for intraoperative surgical guidance and evaluation of surgical margins, thus improving outcomes.[20]

4.2.1. Raman spectroscopy

Raman spectroscopy is a non-invasive technique that can analyse the molecular composition of a tissue, enabling surgeons to identify, examine and determine the quality of the tumour's molecular margins.[145] It is based on the phenomenon that intramolecular bonds cause light to scatter in a manner that is both measurable and predictable, albeit for a very short time constituting <1 part per million of the total reflected light.[145] Point detection techniques can be used to collect molecular information during endoscopy with optical fibre probes, and they have the potential to be extended to imaging.[135] Raman spectroscopy produces inelastic light scattering (returning photons have longer wavelength than the incident photons) and diffuse NIR photons (photons that return after several scattering events and are useful for measuring fine pathological structures) which aid molecular histopathologic examination.[135] It is performed by illuminating tissue with NIR photons that are absorbed by the vibrational/rotational nodes of molecular bonds associated with chemical functional groups specific to mucosal proteins, lipids, and nucleic acids.[135, 225, 226] Some of these photons are then inelastically scattered, forming detailed spectral patterns that can be reduced to the principal components using multivariate statistics. However, the Raman effect is much weaker than fluorescence and can be easily obscured by fluorescence from the tissue or optical fibre itself.[136]

Shim *et al.* demonstrated the use of CCD detector in collecting Raman spectra *in vivo* in the gastrointestinal tract.[227] Molckovsky and colleagues showed that Raman spectroscopy could be used to distinguish between adenomatous and hyperplastic polyps in the colon, with 100% sensitivity, 89% specificity, and 95% accuracy when used *in vivo*.[228] Haka *et al.* used Raman spectroscopy to examine breast tissue *in vivo*, and reported perfect sensitivity and specificity when using their diagnostic algorithm.[229] They highlighted the feasibility of using it for real-time intraoperative margin assessment during partial mastectomy surgery, which could be similarly used for intraoperative margin assessment in HNSCC cases. Stone *et al.* examined biopsy specimens of laryngeal mucosa using Raman spectroscopy and conventional histopathological analysis, and reported 92% sensitivity and 90% specificity for Raman spectra generated over 30 seconds in the diagnosis of invasive cancer (compared to reference spectra generated from histopathologically normal mucosa).[230] In membranous vocal cord specimens, Lau *et al.* reported 69% sensitivity and 94% specificity for invasive carcinoma using Raman spectra recorded over 5 seconds.[231]

Spatially offset Raman spectroscopy (SORS) has been shown to be an effective tool in recovering Raman spectra from up to several millimetres beneath the surface of turbid media.[232] Keller *et al.* found that, using source-detector separations of up to 3.75 mm, SORS can detect sub-millimetre-thick tumours under a 1mm normal layer, and tumours at least 1 mm thick can be detected under a 2 mm normal layer using the Monte Carlo simulation model of breast tumour margin analysis.[232] Other recent developments within Raman spectroscopy include surface enhanced Raman spectroscopy (SERS), coherent anti-Stokes Raman spectroscopy (CARS), and stimulated Raman scatters (SRS),[165, 233] which could all have applications in HNSCC margin analysis. Visualising molecular information using Raman spectroscopy has also been shown to aid in identifying patients with prostate cancer who are at risk of cancer progression from those with no evidence of disease.[234]

Raman spectroscopy provides an objective analysis of the tissue's molecular structure compared to the *ex vivo* histopathological analysis and grading based on tissue morphology. It may provide a more clinically relevant measure of the tumour margin on which to guide surgical excision. It has been possible to stage and grade malignancies from a spectral measurement on the surface of bladder tissue using Raman spectroscopy.[235] Representative reference spectra need to be developed by analysing a large cohort of histologically diagnosed mucosal lesions, against which spectra captured *in vivo* can be compared and leading to algorithms that can quickly produce a diagnosis.[145]

4.2.2. Positron emission tomography and hybrid technologies

PET provides a 3-D image of the functional processes in the body, wherein (18F)-fluorodeoxyglucose (18F-FDG), a glucose analogue, is commonly used as the radiopharmaceutical delivering the positron-emitting radionuclide (tracer), thus reflecting tissue metabolic activity by regional glucose uptake, with cancer cells exhibiting increased use of glucose.[20, 236] 18F-FDG PET highlights metabolic differences between malignant and healthy cells and is the first true molecular imaging modality.[20]A hand-held PET probe to detect high-energy gamma rays during breast cancer surgery has been developed for intra-operative evaluation of tumour localisation and margin status.[162] PET is limited in its use due to high cost, use of ionising radiation, and relatively low spatial resolution (it is difficult to detect small tumours (<1 cm) using this hand-held probe).[20, 136] Since PET on its own provides low anatomical information, it is commonly used in conjunction with CT, and more recently, with MRI which has the advantage of greater soft tissue contrast and fewer artefacts.[14] The PET/MRI hybrid imaging technology combines the functional sequences of MR with the molecular information of PET to provide information about tumour biology and microenvironment [237] – hence the best of both worlds.

A number of studies have evaluated the effectiveness of PET/CT versus PET/MRI in HNSCC. Many studies have found no significant difference between diagnostic capability and anatomic localisation of lesions as detected by both modalities,[238-243] however, there is agreement for tailored use of PET/MRI in the head and neck region since higher soft tissue contrast would aid in diagnosis.[238, 242, 244, 245] Kanda *et al.* found that PET/MRI and PET/CT had equal sensitivities and specificities, and both these were more sensitive compared to MRI alone but less specific, when investigating these modalities in HNSCC.[244] Kubiessa *et al.*[239] showed that PET alone had the highest sensitivity while MRI alone showed best specificity when comparing PET/CT to PET/MRI in patients with HNSCC. Evangelista *et al.* evaluated contrast-enhanced CT (ceCT) with PET in HNSCC cases and found this to be particularly adept at diagnosing small lymph node metastases in positions usually difficult to interpret in the head and neck region.[246] Lee *et al.* found PET/MRI to have acceptable accuracy in T staging compared to endoscopic ultrasound and even higher accuracy (although not statistically significant) than PET/CT in predicting N staging, demonstrating its value as preoperative diagnostic imaging tool in HNSCC.[245] PET/CT has been deemed useful in staging, identification of second primaries, and monitoring in the head and neck region aiding treatment planning.[216, 236, 244, 245, 247]

Hybrid technologies can be used to assess treatment response.[246, 248, 249] Adkins *et al.* found that PET/CT is better than CT in evaluating tumour response to cetuximab in patients with incurable HNSCC.[248] PET/CT has also exhibited high sensitivity to detecting distant metastases, assessing the response to chemotherapy or chemoradiation treatment and in predicting outcome.[246] PET/CT can be used post-therapeutically to assess treatment response, detect residual/recurrent tumours, and exclude distant metastases.[15] "Activatable molecular probes" or "smart" probes may be used to elicit a change in signal upon enzymatic activity or in response to specific biomolecular interactions.[20, 220] These allow very high signal-to-background ratios compared to conventional targeted contrast agents, and lead to the possibility of imaging intracellular targets.[220] Nguyen and Tsien summarise that the use of these fluorescent-labelled molecularly targeted probes would provide real-time, intraoperative distinction of the molecular edge between cancer and adjacent normal tissue, and could aid in discerning and preservation of vital structures such as nerves during surgery.[218] Bhatnagar *et al.* reviewed the use of different PET tracers in hybrid imaging modalities such as PET/CT and PET/MRI to detect and monitor biomarker status to assess effectiveness of therapy in patients with HNSCC.[250] They suggest that treatment strategies could be modulated and adapted by comparing an initial baseline measurement of biomarker expression before treatment to measurements taken during therapy, thus strategically addressing treatment response.[250] Some examples of biomarkers that may be used in this instance are tissue hypoxia, cell proliferation and apoptosis, and epidermal growth factor receptor (EGFR) status.[250] Examples of PET tracers that may be used in relation to biomarkers of response to therapy are described below.

4.2.3. Tumour hypoxia

Hypoxia has been established as an indicator of poor prognosis in HNSCC patients, causing radiation resistance in tumour cells by preventing irreversible damage to DNA by free radicals induced by ionising radiation (oxygen is required for the production of free radicals), thus allowing DNA repair and tumour cell survival.[251, 252] The critical partial pressure of oxygen below which solid tumours resist radiation therapy is about 10-15mm Hg.[252] In comparison, three times the amount of radiation needed to kill tumour cells in normoxic conditions is required to achieve the same in hypoxia. Hypoxia mapping can be performed with the use of molecular imaging to identify tumours that would benefit from hypoxia-reducing treatments.[250]

Fluoromisonidazole (FMISO) has been investigated widely as a PET imaging agent in HNSCC.[253-256] It has been shown that FMISO and FDG uptake do not necessarily correlate, thus representing different tumour properties, with high uptake of FMISO before radiation therapy indicative of locoregional treatment failure and associated poor prognosis.[250, 255, 256] Nevertheless, FMISO may be used in HNSCCs to delineate hypoxic tumour volumes as an indicator to escalate radiation doses.[257-260] The key challenge though is that tumour hypoxia is a dynamic process with a constant change in relative contribution of acute and chronic hypoxia to the total hypoxic volume.[250] One study showed just 46% correlation between two sequential FMISO scans, just 3 days apart, in 20 HNSCC patients.[261] A smaller study with 7 HNSCC patients found correlation between hypoxic volumes on sequential scans in only three patients.[262] Further research is required to investigate the normal variation in FMISO uptake and changes in tumour oxygenation kinetics prior and during therapy, before FMISO imaging can clinically guide hypoxia-mediate intensity modulated radiation therapy (IMRT).[250, 259, 263]

Fluorine 18 fluoroazomycin arabinoside (FAZA) is also a hypoxia-specific PET agent that clears the blood more rapidly than FMISO, thus producing a higher target-to-background signal ratio.[264] Fluorine 18 fluoroerythronitroimidazole (FETNIM) is in theory a stronger indicator of hypoxia than FMISO due to its greater hydrophilia and better pharmacokinetics.[265] Both agents show promise as hypoxia radiotracers, but further research is needed, especially in comparison to FMISO.

Radioactive copper–labelled diacetyl-bis-(N4- methylthiosemicarbazone), or Cu-ATSM, is a neutral lipophilic compound that can permeate cell membranes.[250] In hypoxic conditions, Cu-ATSM molecules are reduced and negatively charged, while they wash out rapidly from normoxic cells, thus selectively accumulating in hypoxic cells resulting in a high SBR.[266] It has been shown that Cu-ATSM showed a significant difference in its uptake in HNSCC patients with residual or recurrent tumour compared to those without, which was not reflected in FDG uptake.[267] Others have shown that Cu-ATSM may be used to identify hypoxic subvolumes for IMRT.[268]

4.2.4. Tumour cell proliferation

While radiation therapy and chemotherapy can lead to a rapid decrease in the rate of cellular proliferation in responding tumours, which precedes a decrease in tumour size, accelerated tumour cell repopulation is an indicator of underlying radiation resistance and hence, treatment failure.[251, 269] Early identification of tumour cell repopulation as part of response assessment through imaging can identify target areas for dose escalation.[250] 3'-Fluoro-3' deoxythymidine (FLT)-PET is used widely to assess cellular proliferation, and unlike FDG, is only taken up by actively dividing cells and not surrounding inflammatory cells, allowing for specific detection of cellular division and subsequent dose escalation in these areas.[270, 271] Changes in the intensity of FLT uptake can be used to reflect cellular response to treatment, even prior to changes in tumour volume.[251, 271] However, FLT does not distinguish between benign and malignant abnormal cervical lymph nodes because its uptake by the germinal centres of reactive lymph nodes leads to a low positive predictive value.[272]

4.2.5. Apoptosis

Chemotherapy and radiation therapy rely on apoptosis to induce tumour cell death. Radiation resistance and treatment failure can result from mutations that lead to uncontrolled cellular

http://dx.doi.org/10.5772/60066

proliferation and dysregulation of apoptotic mechanisms.[273] Technetium 99m (99mTc)–labelled annexin V is a protein that binds to a major phospholipid constituent of cell membranes and has been investigated for imaging apoptosis in various malignancies including HNSCC.[274] The difficulty of radiolabeling annexin V with fluorine 18 has led to the development of other such tracers such as 18F-ML- 10 (2-[5-fluoro-pentyl]-2-methyl-malonic acid) (Aposense; Petach Tikva, Israel). This is a novel small-molecule probe designed to allow visualisation of apoptosis related cellular alterations, useful for differentiating between apoptotic and necrotic cells.[275]

4.2.6. Amino acid transport and protein synthesis

Carbon 11 (11C) methionine is a PET tracer that has been investigated to assess amino acid transport and accelerated protein synthesis in malignant tissue.[276] 11C-methionine allows for effective visualisation of HNSCC, demonstrating a good correlation with FDG demonstrating similar sensitivities and specificities for tumour detection, but does not distinguish between histological grade.[277, 278] It has been shown that there is a decline in 11C-methionine uptake at tumour sites with histology-confirmed complete treatment response in HNSCC patients, in comparison with sites of residual tumour tissue after radiation therapy.[279] Early decrease of 11C-methionine uptake correlates to final tumour volume reduction seen at MRI at the conclusion of treatment in HNSCC patients, suggesting that 11C-methionine can be used for early treatment adaptation.[280] Conversely, Nuutinen *et al.* showed a substantial early decline in 11C-methionine uptake in HNSCC patients after radiation therapy, but the rate of decrease in tracer uptake was comparable between patients with disease recurrence and those with preserved local control.[281] At present, there is no clear role for 11C-methionine in the imaging of HNSCC.[250]

Fluorine 18 fluoroethyltyrosine (FET), an amino acid analogue that is taken up by tumour cells through amino acid transport systems, has shown high diagnostic accuracy in patients with brain tumours, but has lower sensitivity (64-75%) when compared to FDG (89-95%) in the evaluation of HNSCC, making it unsuitable to replace FDG in the initial assessment of HNSCC despite superior specificity (90-100%) than FDG (50-79%).[282-285] FET could still have a role in differentiating between residual tumour tissue and inflammatory tissue after therapy.[250]

4.2.7. Cell membrane synthesis

Choline is incorporated with phospholipids during cell membrane synthesis.[286] A preliminary study[287] using 11C-choline in HNSCC patients found it to be just as effective as FDG for detecting malignant head and neck tumours with PET, however, another study[288] did not find 11C-choline PET/CT to be superior to FDG PET/CT for the detection of recurrent HNSCC.

While this is useful, carcinogenesis and transformation of tissue in HNSCC involves elaborate modification of numerous biomarkers. It would be more useful to assess the overall imbalance in biomarker regulation rather than rely on one marker alone. This considerably complicates the process of molecular diagnosis and analysis through imaging and requires further research.

OFI techniques can be used intraoperatively, in conjunction with information from preoperative MRI, CT or PET, providing a more holistic knowledge of macroscopic and molecular level tissue alterations, enabling ideal surgical guidance.[289-291] This will ultimately improve patient outcome by decreasing MRD in surgical margins.

5. Conclusion

Methods for early detection, molecular assessment of margins and surgical guidance, and assessment of treatment response are instrumental to changing the rate of local recurrence and resultant reduced prognosis in patients with HNSCC by enabling personalised medicine. There are a number of biomarkers that alter expression as tissue transforms. These can be used to assess MRD in surgical margins. Furthermore, optical and molecular imaging techniques can be used to identify molecular changes in biomarker expression, enabling immediate intraoperative decisions on extent of lesion and margin status, reducing the need for repeat surgery and the risk of recurrence. Multimodal imaging will provide more information about diseased tissue, enabling the surgeon to visualise the tumour in terms of its molecular extent and not simply its visual extent (whether with white light or fluorescence). Further research into molecular biomarkers as potential targets for "smart" probes for assessment of MRD in surgical margins is required to enhance current molecular imaging modalities which have applications pre-operatively to delineate lesion location and volume, intra-operatively to assess surgical margins and for surgical guidance, and post-operatively to assess treatment response. Research is also required to assess projected improvements in overall recurrence rates following introduction of these technologies to reveal whether these technologies have improved outcomes in practice.

Author details

Camile S. Farah[1,2*], Keziah John[1] and Jennifer Wu[1]

*Address all correspondence to: camile@oralmedpath.com.au

1 Oral Oncology Research Program, UQ Centre for Clinical Research, The University of Queensland, Herston, Queensland, Australia

2 The Australian Centre for Oral Oncology Research & Education, Brisbane, Queensland, Australia

References

[1] Warnakulasuriya S: Global epidemiology of oral and oropharyngeal cancer. *Oral Oncol* 2009, 45(4-5):309-316.

[2] Alibek K, Kakpenova A, Baiken Y: Role of infectious agents in the carcinogenesis of brain and head and neck cancers. *Infect Agent Cancer* 2013, 8(1):7.

[3] Ferlay J, Shin HR, Bray F, Forman D, Mathers C, Parkin DM: Estimates of worldwide burden of cancer in 2008: GLOBOCAN 2008. *Int J Cancer* 2010, 127(12):2893-2917.

[4] Farah CS, Simanovic B, Dost F: Oral cancer in Australia 1982-2008: a growing need for opportunistic screening and prevention. *Australian dental journal* 2014, 59(3): 349-359.

[5] John K, Wu J, Lee BW, Farah CS: MicroRNAs in Head and Neck Cancer. *International journal of dentistry* 2013, 2013:650218.

[6] Speight PM: Update on oral epithelial dysplasia and progression to cancer. *Head and neck pathology* 2007, 1(1):61-66.

[7] Bhatia N, Lalla Y, Vu AN, Farah CS: Advances in optical adjunctive aids for visualisation and detection of oral malignant and potentially malignant lesions. *International journal of dentistry* 2013, 2013:194029.

[8] Dost F, Le Cao KA, Ford PJ, Farah CS: A retrospective analysis of clinical features of oral malignant and potentially malignant disorders with and without oral epithelial dysplasia. *Oral surgery, oral medicine, oral pathology and oral radiology* 2013, 116(6): 725-733.

[9] Warnakulasuriya S, Johnson NW, van der Waal I: Nomenclature and classification of potentially malignant disorders of the oral mucosa. *J Oral Pathol Med* 2007, 36(10): 575-580.

[10] Dost F, Le Cao K, Ford PJ, Ades C, Farah CS: Malignant transformation of oral epithelial dysplasia: a real-world evaluation of histopathologic grading. *Oral surgery, oral medicine, oral pathology and oral radiology* 2014, 117(3):342-352.

[11] Warnakulasuriya S, Reibel J, Bouquot J, Dabelsteen E: Oral epithelial dysplasia classification systems: predictive value, utility, weaknesses and scope for improvement. *J Oral Pathol Med* 2008, 37(3):127-133.

[12] Lee JJ, Hong WK, Hittelman WN, Mao L, Lotan R, Shin DM, Benner SE, Xu XC, Lee JS, Papadimitrakopoulou VM *et al*: Predicting cancer development in oral leukoplakia: ten years of translational research. *Clin Cancer Res* 2000, 6(5):1702-1710.

[13] Cervigne NK, Reis PP, Machado J, Sadikovic B, Bradley G, Galloni NN, Pintilie M, Jurisica I, Perez-Ordonez B, Gilbert R *et al*: Identification of a microRNA signature associated with progression of leukoplakia to oral carcinoma. *Hum Mol Genet* 2009, 18(24):4818-4829.

[14] Farah C, Bhatia N, John K, Lee B: Minimum intervention dentistry in oral medicine. *Australian dental journal* 2013, 58 Suppl 1:85-94.

[15] Tantiwongkosi B, Yu F, Kanard A, Miller FR: Role of F-FDG PET/CT in pre and post treatment evaluation in head and neck carcinoma. *World journal of radiology* 2014, 6(5):177-191.

[16] Gillison ML, Castellsague X, Chaturvedi A, Goodman MT, Snijders P, Tommasino M, Arbyn M, Franceschi S: Eurogin 2012 roadmap: Comparative epidemiology of HPV infection and associated cancers of the head and neck and cervix. *Int J Cancer* 2013, 134(3):497-507.

[17] Heuveling DA, de Bree R, van Dongen GA: The potential role of non-FDG-PET in the management of head and neck cancer. *Oral Oncol* 2011, 47(1):2-7.

[18] Nagadia R, Pandit P, Coman WB, Cooper-White J, Punyadeera C: miRNAs in head and neck cancer revisited. *Cell Oncol* 2013, 36(1):1-7.

[19] de Carvalho AC, Kowalski LP, Campos AH, Soares FA, Carvalho AL, Vettore AL: Clinical significance of molecular alterations in histologically negative surgical margins of head and neck cancer patients. *Oral Oncol* 2012, 48(3):240-248.

[20] Hussain T, Nguyen QT: Molecular imaging for cancer diagnosis and surgery. *Advanced drug delivery reviews* 2014, 66:90-100.

[21] Eckardt A, Barth EL, Kokemueller H, Wegener G: Recurrent carcinoma of the head and neck: treatment strategies and survival analysis in a 20-year period. *Oral Oncol* 2004, 40(4):427-432.

[22] Karim-Kos HE, de Vries E, Soerjomataram I, Lemmens V, Siesling S, Coebergh JWW: Recent trends of cancer in Europe: A combined approach of incidence, survival and mortality for 17 cancer sites since the 1990s. *Eur J Cancer* 2008, 44(10):1345-1389.

[23] Slootweg PJ, Hordijk GJ, Schade Y, van Es RJJ, Koole R: Treatment failure and margin status in head and neck cancer. A critical view on the potential value of molecular pathology. *Oral Oncol* 2002, 38(5):500-503.

[24] Braakhuis BJ, Bloemena E, Leemans CR, Brakenhoff RH: Molecular analysis of surgical margins in head and neck cancer: more than a marginal issue. *Oral Oncol* 2010, 46(7):485-491.

[25] Woolgar JA, Triantafyllou A: A histopathological appraisal of surgical margins in oral and oropharyngeal cancer resection specimens. *Oral Oncol* 2005, 41(10):1034-1043.

[26] Lyons A: Current concepts in the management of oral cancer. *Dental update* 2006, 33(9):538-539, 542-535.

[27] Gandour-Edwards RF, Donald PJ, Lie JT: Clinical utility of intraoperative frozen-section diagnosis in head and neck-surgery - a quality assurance perspective. *Head Neck* 1993, 15(5):373-376.

[28] Gandour-Edwards RF, Donald PJ, Wiese DA: Accuracy of intraoperative frozen section diagnosis in head and neck-surgery - experience at a university medical-center. *Head Neck* 1993, 15(1):33-38.

[29] Laccourreye O, Hans S, Menard M, Garcia D, Brasnu D, Holsinger C: Transoral lateral oropharyngectomy for squamous cell carcinoma of the tonsillar region - II. An analysis of the incidence, related variables, and consequences of local recurrence. *Arch Otolaryngol Head Neck Surg* 2005, 131(7):592-599.

[30] Spiro RH, Guillamondegui O, Paulino AF, Huvos AG: Pattern of invasion and margin assessment in patients with oral tongue cancer. *Head Neck* 1999, 21(5):408-413.

[31] Slaughter DP, Southwick HW, Smejkal W: Field cancerization in oral stratified squamous epithelium: Clinical implication of multicentric origin. *Cancer* 1953, 6(5): 963-968.

[32] Wong LS, McMahon J, Devine J, McLellan D, Thompson E, Farrow A, Moos K, Ayoub A: Influence of close resection margins on local recurrence and disease-specific survival in oral and oropharyngeal carcinoma. *Br J Oral Maxillofac Surg* 2012, 50(2): 102-108.

[33] Nason RW, Binahmed A, Pathak KA, Abdoh AA, Sandor GKB: What is the adequate margin of surgical resection in oral cancer? *Oral Surg Oral Med Oral Pathol Oral Radiol Endod* 2009, 107(5):625-629.

[34] Goldenberg D, Harden S, Masayesva BG, Ha P, Benoit N, Westra WH, Koch WM, Sidransky D, Califano JA: Intraoperative molecular margin analysis in head and neck cancer. *Arch Otolaryngol Head Neck Surg* 2004, 130(1):39-44.

[35] Partridge M, Li SR, Pateromichelakis S, Francis R, Phillips E, Huang XH, Tesfa-Selase F, Langdon JD: Detection of minimal residual cancer to investigate why oral tumors recur despite seemingly adequate treatment. *Clin Cancer Res* 2000, 6(7):2718-2725.

[36] Yanamoto S, Yamada S, Takahashi H, Yoshitomi I, Kawasaki G, Ikeda H, Minamizato T, Shiraishi T, Fujita S, Ikeda T *et al*: Clinicopathological risk factors for local recurrence in oral squamous cell carcinoma. *International journal of oral and maxillofacial surgery* 2012, 41(10):1195-1200.

[37] Ha PK, Benoit NE, Yochem R, Sciubba J, Zahurak M, Sidransky D, Pevsner J, Westra WH, Califano J: A transcriptional progression model for head and neck cancer. *Clin Cancer Res* 2003, 9(8):3058-3064.

[38] Smith J, Rattay T, McConkey C, Helliwell T, Mehanna H: Biomarkers in dysplasia of the oral cavity: a systematic review. *Oral Oncol* 2009, 45(8):647-653.

[39] Pitiyage G, Tilakaratne WM, Tavassoli M, Warnakulasuriya S: Molecular markers in oral epithelial dysplasia: review. *J Oral Pathol Med* 2009, 38(10):737-752.

[40] Tabor MP, Braakhuis BJ, van der Wal JE, van Diest PJ, Leemans CR, Brakenhoff RH, Kummer JA: Comparative molecular and histological grading of epithelial dysplasia of the oral cavity and the oropharynx. *J Pathol* 2003, 199(3):354-360.

[41] Egger G, Liang G, Aparicio A, Jones PA: Epigenetics in human disease and prospects for epigenetic therapy. *Nature* 2004, 429(6990):457-463.

[42] Gasche JA, Goel A: Epigenetic mechanisms in oral carcinogenesis. *Future oncology (London, England)* 2012, 8(11):1407-1425.

[43] Feinberg AP, Ohlsson R, Henikoff S: The epigenetic progenitor origin of human cancer. *Nature reviews Genetics* 2006, 7(1):21-33.

[44] Nagpal JK, Das BR: Oral cancer: reviewing the present understanding of its molecular mechanism and exploring the future directions for its effective management. *Oral Oncol* 2003, 39(3):213-221.

[45] Lingen MW, Pinto A, Mendes RA, Franchini R, Czerninski R, Tilakaratne WM, Partridge M, Peterson DE, Woo SB: Genetics/epigenetics of oral premalignancy: current status and future research. *Oral diseases* 2011, 17 Suppl 1:7-22.

[46] Santhi WS, Sebastian P, Varghese BT, Prakash O, Pillai MR: NF-kappaB and COX-2 during oral tumorigenesis and in assessment of minimal residual disease in surgical margins. *Experimental and molecular pathology* 2006, 81(2):123-130.

[47] Santhi WS, Prathibha R, Charles S, Anurup KG, Reshmi G, Ramachandran S, Jissa VT, Sebastian P, Radhakrishna Pillai M: Oncogenic microRNAs as biomarkers of oral tumorigenesis and minimal residual disease. *Oral Oncol* 2013, 49(6):567-575.

[48] Cruz IB, Meijer C, Snijders PJF, Snow GB, Walboomers JMM, van der Waal I: p53 immunoexpression in non-malignant oral mucosa adjacent to oral squamous cell carcinoma: potential consequences for clinical management. *J Pathol* 2000, 191(2):132-137.

[49] Bilde A, von Buchwald C, Dabelsteen E, Therkildsen MH, Dabelsteen S: Molecular markers in the surgical margin of oral carcinomas. *J Oral Pathol Med* 2009, 38(1):72-78.

[50] Bergshoeff VE, Hopman AHN, Zwijnenberg IR, Ramaekers FCS, Bot FJ, Kremer B, Manni JJ, Speel EJM: Chromosome instability in resection margins predicts recurrence of oral squamous cell carcinoma. *J Pathol* 2008, 215(3):347-348.

[51] Tunca B, Erisen L, Coskun H, Cecener G, Ozuysal S, Egeli U: p53 gene mutations in surgical margins and primary tumor tissues of patients with squamous cell carcinoma of the head and neck. *Tumori* 2007, 93(2):182-188.

[52] Graveland AP, Golusinski PJ, Buijze M, Douma R, Sons N, Kuik DJ, Bloemena E, Leemans CR, Brakenhoff RH, Braakhuis BJ: Loss of heterozygosity at 9p and p53 immunopositivity in surgical margins predict local relapse in head and neck squamous cell carcinoma. *Int J Cancer* 2011, 128(8):1852-1859.

[53] Graveland AP, Bremmer JF, de Maaker M, Brink A, Cobussen P, Zwart M, Braakhuis BJ, Bloemena E, van der Waal I, Leemans CR *et al*: Molecular screening of oral precancer. *Oral Oncol* 2013, 49(12):1129-1135.

[54] Nathan CAO, Amirghahri N, Rice C, Abreo FW, Shi RH, Stucker FJ: Molecular analysis of surgical margins in head and neck squamous cell carcinoma patients. *Laryngoscope* 2002, 112(12):2129-2140.

[55] Martone T, Gillio-Tos A, De Marco L, Fiano V, Maule M, Cavalot A, Garzaro M, Merletti F, Cortesina G: Association between hypermethylated tumor and paired surgical margins in head and neck squamous cell carcinomas. *Clin Cancer Res* 2007, 13(17): 5089-5094.

[56] Sinha P, Bahadur S, Thakar A, Matta A, Macha M, Ralhan R, Gupta SD: Significance of promoter hypermethylation of p16 gene for margin assessment in carcinoma tongue. *Head Neck* 2009, 31(11):1423-1430.

[57] Wong TS, Man MW, Lam AK, Wei WI, Kwong YL, Yuen AP: The study of p16 and p15 gene methylation in head and neck squamous cell carcinoma and their quantitative evaluation in plasma by real-time PCR. *Eur J Cancer* 2003, 39(13):1881-1887.

[58] Nathan CAO, Franklin S, Abreo FW, Nassar R, De Benedetti A, Glass J: Analysis of surgical margins with the molecular marker eIF4E: A prognostic factor in patients with head and neck cancer. *J Clin Oncol* 1999, 17(9):2909-2914.

[59] Tan HK, Saulnier P, Auperin A, Lacroix L, Casiraghi O, Janot F, Fouret P, Temam S: Quantitative methylation analyses of resection margins predict local recurrences and disease-specific deaths in patients with head and neck squamous cell carcinomas. *BrJ Cancer* 2008, 99(2):357-363.

[60] Roh JL, Westra WH, Califano JA, Sidransky D, Koch WM: Tissue imprint for molecular mapping of deep surgical margins in patients with head and neck squamous cell carcinoma. *Head Neck* 2012, 34(11):1529-1536.

[61] Supic G, Kozomara R, Jovic N, Zeljic K, Magic Z: Prognostic significance of tumor-related genes hypermethylation detected in cancer-free surgical margins of oral squamous cell carcinomas. *Oral Oncol* 2011, 47(8):702-708.

[62] Ott CE, Skroch E, Steinhart H, Verdorfer I, Pahl S, Iro H, Gebhart E, Bohlender JE: Thin section arrays for I-FISH analysis of chromosome-specific imbalances in squamous cell carcinomas of the head and neck. *Int J Oncol* 2002, 20(3):623-630.

[63] Bremmer JF, Braakhuis BJM, Brink A, Broeckaert MAM, Belien JAM, Meijer GA, Kuik DJ, Leemans CR, Bloemena E, van der Waal I *et al*: Comparative evaluation of genetic assays to identify oral pre-cancerous fields. *J Oral Pathol Med* 2008, 37(10): 599-606.

[64] Stafford ND, Ashman JNE, MacDonald AW, Ell SR, Monson JRT, Greenman J: Genetic analysis of head and neck squamous cell carcinoma and surrounding mucosa. *Arch Otolaryngol Head Neck Surg* 1999, 125(12):1341-1348.

[65] Preuss SF, Brieger J, Essig EK, Stenzel MJ, Mann WJ: Quantitative DNA measurement in oropharyngeal squamous cell carcinoma and surrounding mucosa. *ORL J Otorhinolaryngol Relat Spec* 2004, 66(6):320-324.

[66] Szukala K, Sowinska A, Wierzbicka M, Biczysko W, Szyfter W, Szyfter K: Does loss of heterozygosity in critical genome regions predict a local relapse in patients after laryngectomy? *Mutat Res* 2006, 600(1-2):67-76.

[67] Brieger J, Kastner J, Gosepath J, Mann WJ: Evaluation of microsatellite amplifications at chromosomal locus 3q26 as surrogate marker for premalignant changes in mucosa surrounding head and neck squamous cell carcinoma. *Cancer Genet Cytogenet* 2006, 167(1):26-31.

[68] Poh CF, Zhang L, Anderson DW, Durham JS, Williams RM, Priddy RW, Berean KW, Ng S, Tseng OL, MacAulay C *et al*: Fluorescence visualization detection of field alterations in tumor margins of oral cancer patients. *Clin Cancer Res* 2006, 12(22): 6716-6722.

[69] Mascolo M, Siano M, Ilardi G, Russo D, Merolla F, De Rosa G, Staibano S: Epigenetic disregulation in oral cancer. *International journal of molecular sciences* 2012, 13(2): 2331-2353.

[70] Roh J-L, Wang XV, Manola J, Sidransky D, Forastiere AA, Koch WM: Clinical correlates of promoter hypermethylation of four target genes in head and neck cancer: A cooperative group correlative study. *Clin Cancer Res* 2013, 19(9):2528-2540.

[71] Perez-Sayans M, Suarez-Penaranda JM, Gayoso-Diz P, Barros-Angueira F, Gandara-Rey JM, Garcia-Garcia A: p16(INK4a)/CDKN2 expression and its relationship with oral squamous cell carcinoma is our current knowledge enough? *Cancer letters* 2011, 306(2):134-141.

[72] Kato K, Hara A, Kuno T, Mori H, Yamashita T, Toida M, Shibata T: Aberrant promoter hypermethylation of p16 and MGMT genes in oral squamous cell carcinomas and the surrounding normal mucosa. *Journal of cancer research and clinical oncology* 2006, 132(11):735-743.

[73] Rainsbury JW, Ahmed W, Williams HK, Roberts S, Paleri V, Mehanna H: Prognostic biomarkers of survival in oropharyngeal squamous cell carcinoma: systematic review and meta-analysis. *Head Neck* 2013, 35(7):1048-1055.

[74] Califano J, Westra WH, Meininger G, Corio R, Koch WM, Sidransky D: Genetic progression and clonal relationship of recurrent premalignant head and neck lesions. *Clin Cancer Res* 2000, 6(2):347-352.

[75] Sidransky D: Molecular markers in cancer diagnosis. *Journal of the National Cancer Institute Monographs* 1995(17):27-29.

[76] Mao L, Lee JS, Fan YH, Ro JY, Batsakis JG, Lippman S, Hittelman W, Hong WK: Frequent microsatellite alterations at chromosomes 9p21 and 3p14 in oral premalignant lesions and their value in cancer risk assessment. *Nature medicine* 1996, 2(6):682-685.

[77] Lippman SM, Sudbo J, Hong WK: Oral cancer prevention and the evolution of molecular-targeted drug development. *J Clin Oncol* 2005, 23(2):346-356.

[78] Hong WK, Spitz MR, Lippman SM: Cancer chemoprevention in the 21st century: genetics, risk modeling, and molecular targets. *J Clin Oncol* 2000, 18(21 Suppl):9S-18S.

[79] Califano J, van der Riet P, Westra W, Nawroz H, Clayman G, Piantadosi S, Corio R, Lee D, Greenberg B, Koch W *et al*: Genetic progression model for head and neck cancer: implications for field cancerization. *Cancer Res* 1996, 56(11):2488-2492.

[80] Sidransky D: Molecular genetics of head and neck cancer. *Current opinion in oncology* 1995, 7(3):229-233.

[81] Tsui IF, Rosin MP, Zhang L, Ng RT, Lam WL: Multiple aberrations of chromosome 3p detected in oral premalignant lesions. *Cancer Prev Res (Phila)* 2008, 1(6):424-429.

[82] Tabor MP, Brakenhoff RH, van Houten VM, Kummer JA, Snel MH, Snijders PJ, Snow GB, Leemans CR, Braakhuis BJ: Persistence of genetically altered fields in head and neck cancer patients: biological and clinical implications. *Clin Cancer Res* 2001, 7(6): 1523-1532.

[83] Partridge M, Pateromichelakis S, Phillips E, Emilion GG, A'Hern RP, Langdon JD: A case-control study confirms that microsatellite assay can identify patients at risk of developing oral squamous cell carcinoma within a field of cancerization. *Cancer Res* 2000, 60(14):3893-3898.

[84] Rosin MP, Cheng X, Poh C, Lam WL, Huang Y, Lovas J, Berean K, Epstein JB, Priddy R, Le ND *et al*: Use of allelic loss to predict malignant risk for low-grade oral epithelial dysplasia. *Clin Cancer Res* 2000, 6(2):357-362.

[85] Rosin MP, Lam WL, Poh C, Le ND, Li RJ, Zeng T, Priddy R, Zhang L: 3p14 and 9p21 loss is a simple tool for predicting second oral malignancy at previously treated oral cancer sites. *Cancer Res* 2002, 62(22):6447-6450.

[86] Sardi I, Franchi A, Ferriero G, Frittelli A, Bruschini L, Montali E, Gallo O: Prediction of recurrence by microsatellite analysis in head and neck cancer. *Genes Chromosomes Cancer* 2000, 29(3):201-206.

[87] Zhang L, Poh CF, Williams M, Laronde DM, Berean K, Gardner PJ, Jiang H, Wu L, Lee JJ, Rosin MP: Loss of heterozygosity (LOH) profiles--validated risk predictors for progression to oral cancer. *Cancer Prev Res (Phila)* 2012, 5(9):1081-1089.

[88] Lingen MW, Szabo E: Validation of LOH profiles for assessing oral cancer risk. *Cancer Prev Res (Phila)* 2012, 5(9):1075-1077.

[89] Chin D, Boyle GM, Theile DR, Parsons PG, Coman WB: Molecular introduction to head and neck cancer (HNSCC) carcinogenesis. *British journal of plastic surgery* 2004, 57(7):595-602.

[90] Choi S, Myers JN: Molecular pathogenesis of oral squamous cell carcinoma: implications for therapy. *Journal of dental research* 2008, 87(1):14-32.

[91] Kim MM, Califano JA: Molecular pathology of head-and-neck cancer. *Int J Cancer* 2004, 112(4):545-553.

[92] Mirzayans R, Andrais B, Scott A, Murray D: New insights into p53 signaling and cancer cell response to DNA damage: implications for cancer therapy. *Journal of biomedicine & biotechnology* 2012, 2012:170325.

[93] Brennan JA, Mao L, Hruban RH, Boyle JO, Eby YJ, Koch WM, Goodman SN, Sidransky D: Molecular assessment of histopathological staging in squamous-cell carcinoma of the head and neck. *N Engl J Med* 1995, 332(7):429-435.

[94] van Houten VMM, Tabor MP, van den Brekel MWM, Kummer JA, Denkers F, Dijkstra J, Leemans R, van der Waal I, Snow GB, Brakenhoff RH: Mutated p53 as a molecular marker for the diagnosis of head and neck cancer. *J Pathol* 2002, 198(4):476-486.

[95] Pena Murillo C, Huang X, Hills A, McGurk M, Lyons A, Jeannon JP, Odell E, Brown A, Lavery K, Barrett W *et al*: The utility of molecular diagnostics to predict recurrence of head and neck carcinoma. *Br J Cancer* 2012, 107(7):1138-1143.

[96] Yi HJ, Zhang BQ, Guo W, Zhao LD, Yang SM: The role of molecular margins as prognostic factors in laryngeal carcinoma in Chinese patients. *Acta oto-laryngologica* 2012, 132(8):874-878.

[97] van Houten VMM, Leemans CR, Kummer JA, Dijkstra J, Kuik DJ, van den Brekel MWM, Snow GB, Brakenhoff RH: Molecular diagnosis of surgical margins and local recurrence in head and neck cancer patients: A prospective study. *Clin Cancer Res* 2004, 10(11):3614-3620.

[98] Warnakulasuriya S: Lack of molecular markers to predict malignant potential of oral precancer. *J Pathol* 2000, 190(4):407-409.

[99] Cruz IB, Snijders PJ, Meijer CJ, Braakhuis BJ, Snow GB, Walboomers JM, van der Waal I: p53 expression above the basal cell layer in oral mucosa is an early event of malignant transformation and has predictive value for developing oral squamous cell carcinoma. *J Pathol* 1998, 184(4):360-368.

[100] Hall GL, Shaw RJ, Field EA, Rogers SN, Sutton DN, Woolgar JA, Lowe D, Liloglou T, Field JK, Risk JM: p16 Promoter methylation is a potential predictor of malignant transformation in oral epithelial dysplasia. *Cancer epidemiology, biomarkers & preven-*

tion : a publication of the American Association for Cancer Research, cosponsored by the American Society of Preventive Oncology 2008, 17(8):2174-2179.

[101] Bradley G, Odell EW, Raphael S, Ho J, Le LW, Benchimol S, Kamel-Reid S: Abnormal DNA content in oral epithelial dysplasia is associated with increased risk of progression to carcinoma. *Br J Cancer* 2010, 103(9):1432-1442.

[102] Poeta ML, Manola J, Goldwasser MA, Forastiere A, Benoit N, Califano JA, Ridge JA, Goodwin J, Kenady D, Saunders J *et al*: TP53 mutations and survival in squamous-cell carcinoma of the head and neck. *N Engl J Med* 2007, 357(25):2552-2561.

[103] Van der Vorst S, Dekairelle AF, Weynand B, Hamoir M, Gala JL: Assessment of p53 functional activity in tumor cells and histologically normal mucosa from patients with head and neck squamous cell carcinoma. *Head Neck* 2012, 34(11):1542-1550.

[104] Vered M, Allon I, Dayan D: Maspin, p53, p63, and Ki-67 in epithelial lesions of the tongue: from hyperplasia through dysplasia to carcinoma. *J Oral Pathol Med* 2009, 38(3):314-320.

[105] Bortoluzzi MC, Yurgel LS, Dekker NP, Jordan RC, Regezi JA: Assessment of p63 expression in oral squamous cell carcinomas and dysplasias. *Oral Surg Oral Med Oral Pathol Oral Radiol Endod* 2004, 98(6):698-704.

[106] Murti PR, Warnakulasuriya KA, Johnson NW, Bhonsle RB, Gupta PC, Daftary DK, Mehta FS: p53 expression in oral precancer as a marker for malignant potential. *J Oral Pathol Med* 1998, 27(5):191-196.

[107] Nasser W, Flechtenmacher C, Holzinger D, Hofele C, Bosch FX: Aberrant expression of p53, p16INK4a and Ki-67 as basic biomarker for malignant progression of oral leukoplakias. *J Oral Pathol Med* 2011, 40(8):629-635.

[108] Nathan CO, Liu L, Li BD, Abreo FW, Nandy I, De Benedetti A: Detection of the proto-oncogene eIF4E in surgical margins may predict recurrence in head and neck cancer. *Oncogene* 1997, 15(5):579-584.

[109] Sunavala-Dossabhoy G, Palaniyandi S, Clark C, Nathan CO, Abreo FW, Caldito G: Analysis of eIF4E and 4EBP1 mRNAs in head and neck cancer. *Laryngoscope* 2011, 121(10):2136-2141.

[110] Nathan CAO, Sanders K, Abreo FW, Nassar R, Glass J: Correlation of p53 and the proto-oncogene eIF4E in larynx cancers: Prognostic implications. *Cancer Res* 2000, 60(13):3599-3604.

[111] Chen YK, Hsue SS, Lin LM: Expression of p63 protein and mRNA in oral epithelial dysplasia. *J Oral Pathol Med* 2005, 34(4):232-239.

[112] Takeda T, Sugihara K, Hirayama Y, Hirano M, Tanuma JI, Semba I: Immunohistological evaluation of Ki-67, p63, CK19 and p53 expression in oral epithelial dysplasias. *J Oral Pathol Med* 2006, 35(6):369-375.

[113] Choi HR, Tucker SA, Huang Z, Gillenwater AM, Luna MA, Batsakis JG, El-Naggar AK: Differential expressions of cyclin-dependent kinase inhibitors (p27 and p21) and their relation to p53 and Ki-67 in oral squamous tumorigenesis. *Int J Oncol* 2003, 22(2):409-414.

[114] Calin GA, Croce CM: MicroRNA signatures in human cancers. *Nat Rev Cancer* 2006, 6(11):857-866.

[115] Clague J, Lippman SM, Yang H, Hildebrandt MA, Ye Y, Lee JJ, Wu X: Genetic variation in microRNA genes and risk of oral premalignant lesions. *Molecular carcinogenesis* 2010, 49(2):183-189.

[116] Gorenchtein M, Poh CF, Saini R, Garnis C: MicroRNAs in an oral cancer context - from basic biology to clinical utility. *Journal of dental research* 2012, 91(5):440-446.

[117] Barker EV, Cervigne NK, Reis PP, Goswami RS, Xu W, Weinreb I, Irish JC, Kamel-Reid S: MicroRNA evaluation of unknown primary lesions in the head and neck. *Mol Cancer* 2009, 8.

[118] Malumbres M: miRNAs and cancer: An epigenetics view. *Molecular aspects of medicine* 2012, 34(4):863-874.

[119] Wu BH, Xiong XP, Jia J, Zhang WF: MicroRNAs: new actors in the oral cancer scene. *Oral Oncol* 2011, 47(5):314-319.

[120] Perez-Sayans M, Pilar GD, Barros-Angueira F, Suarez-Penaranda JM, Fernandez AC, Gandara-Rey JM, Garcia-Garcia A: Current trends in miRNAs and their relationship with oral squamous cell carcinoma. *J Oral Pathol Med* 2012, 41(6):433-443.

[121] Scapoli L, Palmieri A, Lo Muzio L, Pezzetti F, Rubini C, Girardi A, Farinella F, Mazzotta M, Carinci F: MicroRNA expression profiling of oral carcinoma identifies new markers of tumor progression. *International journal of immunopathology and pharmacology* 2010, 23(4):1229-1234.

[122] Calin GA, Dumitru CD, Shimizu M, Bichi R, Zupo S, Noch E, Aldler H, Rattan S, Keating M, Rai K *et al*: Frequent deletions and down-regulation of micro- RNA genes miR15 and miR16 at 13q14 in chronic lymphocytic leukemia. *Proc Natl Acad Sci U S A* 2002, 99(24):15524-15529.

[123] Calin GA, Sevignani C, Dan Dumitru C, Hyslop T, Noch E, Yendamuri S, Shimizu M, Rattan S, Bullrich F, Negrini M *et al*: Human microRNA genes are frequently located at fragile sites and genomic regions involved in cancers. *Proc Natl Acad Sci U S A* 2004, 101(9):2999-3004.

[124] Childs G, Fazzari M, Kung G, Kawachi N, Brandwein-Gensler M, McLemore M, Chen Q, Burk RD, Smith RV, Prystowsky MB *et al*: Low-level expression of microRNAs let-7d and mir-205 are prognostic markers of head and neck squamous cell carcinoma. *Am J Pathol* 2009, 174(3):736-745.

[125] Kozaki K-i, Imoto I, Mogi S, Omura K, Inazawa J: Exploration of tumor-suppressive microRNAs silenced by DNA hypermethylation in oral cancer. *Cancer Res* 2008, 68(7): 2094-2105.

[126] Li J, Huang H, Sun L, Yang M, Pan C, Chen W, Wu D, Lin Z, Zeng C, Yao Y *et al*: miR-21 indicates poor prognosis in tongue squamous cell carcinomas as an apoptosis inhibitor. *Clin Cancer Res* 2009, 15(12):3998-4008.

[127] Lajer CB, Garnaes E, Friis-Hansen L, Norrild B, Therkildsen MH, Glud M, Rossing M, Lajer H, Svane D, Skotte L *et al*: The role of miRNAs in human papilloma virus (HPV)-associated cancers: bridging between HPV-related head and neck cancer and cervical cancer. *Br J Cancer* 2012, 106(9):1526-1534.

[128] Lajer CB, Nielsen FC, Friis-Hansen L, Norrild B, Borup R, Garnaes E, Rossing M, Specht L, Therkildsen MH, Nauntofte B *et al*: Different miRNA signatures of oral and pharyngeal squamous cell carcinomas: a prospective translational study. *Br J Cancer* 2011, 104(5):830-840.

[129] Zhang X, Cairns M, Rose B, O'Brien C, Shannon K, Clark J, Gamble J, Tran N: Alterations in miRNA processing and expression in pleomorphic adenomas of the salivary gland. *Int J Cancer* 2009, 124(12):2855-2863.

[130] Reis PP, Tomenson M, Cervigne NK, Machado J, Jurisica I, Pintilie M, Sukhai MA, Perez-Ordonez B, Grenman R, Gilbert RW *et al*: Programmed cell death 4 loss increases tumor cell invasion and is regulated by miR-21 in oral squamous cell carcinoma. *Mol Cancer* 2010, 9:238.

[131] Zheng ZM, Wang X: Regulation of cellular miRNA expression by human papillomaviruses. *Biochim Biophys Acta* 2011, 1809(11-12):668-677.

[132] Babu JM, Prathibha R, Jijith VS, Hariharan R, Pillai MR: A miR-centric view of head and neck cancers. *Biochim Biophys Acta* 2011, 1816(1):67-72.

[133] Langevin SM, Stone RA, Bunker CH, Grandis JR, Sobol RW, Taioli E: MicroRNA-137 promoter methylation in oral rinses from patients with squamous cell carcinoma of the head and neck is associated with gender and body mass index. *Carcinogenesis* 2010, 31(5):864-870.

[134] Xiao W, Bao ZX, Zhang CY, Zhang XY, Shi LJ, Zhou ZT, Jiang WW: Upregulation of miR-31* is negatively associated with recurrent/newly formed oral leukoplakia. *PLoS One* 2012, 7(6):1-10.

[135] Wang TD, Van Dam J: Optical biopsy: a new frontier in endoscopic detection and diagnosis. *Clin Gastroenterol Hepatol* 2004, 2(9):744-753.

[136] Keereweer S, Kerrebijn JD, van Driel PB, Xie B, Kaijzel EL, Snoeks TJ, Que I, Hutteman M, van der Vorst JR, Mieog JS *et al*: Optical image-guided surgery--where do we stand? *Mol Imaging Biol* 2011, 13(2):199-207.

[137] Zhu Y, Terry NG, Wax A: Angle-resolved low-coherence interferometry: An optical biopsy technique for clinical detection of dysplasia in Barretts esophagus. *Expert Review of Gastroenterology and Hepatology* 2012, 6(1):37-41.

[138] Hamdoon Z, Jerjes W, Upile T, McKenzie G, Jay A, Hopper C: Optical coherence tomography in the assessment of suspicious oral lesions: An immediate ex vivo study. *Photodiagnosis and Photodynamic Therapy* 2013, 10(1):17-27.

[139] Adhi M, Duker JS: Optical coherence tomography-current and future applications. *Curr Opin Ophthalmol* 2013, 24(3):213-221.

[140] Whiteman SC, Yang Y, Gey van Pittius D, Stephens M, Parmer J, Spiteri MA: Optical coherence tomography: real-time imaging of bronchial airways microstructure and detection of inflammatory/neoplastic morphologic changes. *Clin Cancer Res* 2006, 12(3 Pt 1):813-818.

[141] Lee CK, Tsai MT, Lee HC, Chen HM, Chiang CP, Wang YM, Yang CC: Diagnosis of oral submucous fibrosis with optical coherence tomography. *J Biomed Opt* 2009, 14(5): 054008.

[142] Ozawa N, Sumi Y, Shimozato K, Chong C, Kurabayashi T: In vivo imaging of human labial glands using advanced optical coherence tomography. *Oral Surg Oral Med Oral Pathol Oral Radiol Endod* 2009, 108(3):425-429.

[143] Fujimoto JG: Optical coherence tomography for ultrahigh resolution in vivo imaging. *Nature Biotechnol* 2003, 21(11):1361-1367.

[144] Brezinski ME, Tearney GJ, Boppart SA, Swanson EA, Southern JF, Fujimoto JG: Optical biopsy with optical coherence tomography: Feasibility for surgical diagnostics. *J Surg Res* 1997, 71(1):32-40.

[145] Hughes OR, Stone N, Kraft M, Arens C, Birchall MA: Optical and molecular techniques to identify tumor margins within the larynx. *Head Neck* 2010, 32(11):1544-1553.

[146] Hamdoon Z, Jerjes W, Al-Delayme R, McKenzie G, Jay A, Hopper C: Structural validation of oral mucosal tissue using optical coherence tomography. *Head and Neck Oncology* 2012, 4(1).

[147] Jerjes W, Upile T, Conn B, Hamdoon Z, Betz CS, McKenzie G, Radhi H, Vourvachis M, El Maaytah M, Sandison A *et al*: In vitro examination of suspicious oral lesions using optical coherence tomography. *British Journal of Oral and Maxillofacial Surgery* 2010, 48(1):18-25.

[148] Savastru D, Chang EW, Miclos S, Pitman MB, Patel A, Iftimia N: Detection of breast surgical margins with optical coherence tomography imaging: a concept evaluation study. *J Biomed Opt* 2014, 19(5):056001.

[149] South FA, Chaney EJ, Marjanovic M, Adie SG, Boppart SA: Differentiation of ex vivo human breast tissue using polarization-sensitive optical coherence tomography. *Biomed Opt Express* 2014, 5(10):3417-3426.

[150] Alawi SA, Kuck M, Wahrlich C, Batz S, McKenzie G, Fluhr JW, Lademann J, Ulrich M: Optical coherence tomography for presurgical margin assessment of non-melanoma skin cancer - a practical approach. *Exp Dermatol* 2013, 22(8):547-551.

[151] Pelosini L, Smith HB, Schofield JB, Meeckings A, Dhital A, Khandwala M: In vivo optical coherence tomography (OCT) in periocular basal cell carcinoma: correlations between in vivo OCT images and postoperative histology. *Br J Ophthalmol* 2013, 97(7): 890-894.

[152] Wessels R, van Beurden M, de Bruin DM, Faber DJ, Vincent AD, Sanders J, van Leeuwen TG, Ruers TJ: The value of optical coherence tomography in determining surgical margins in squamous cell carcinoma of the vulva: a single-center prospective study. *Int J Gynecol Cancer* 2014.

[153] Skarecky DW, Brenner M, Rajan S, Rodriguez E, Jr., Narula N, Melgoza F, Ahlering TE: Zero positive surgical margins after radical prostatectomy: is the end in sight. *Expert Rev Med Devices* 2008, 5(6):709-717.

[154] Pyhtila JW, Chalut KJ, Boyer JD, Keener J, D'Amico T, Gottfried M, Gress F, Wax A: In situ detection of nuclear atypia in Barrett's esophagus by using angle-resolved low-coherence interferometry. *Gastrointest Endosc* 2007, 65(3):487-491.

[155] Terry NG, Zhu Y, Rinehart MT, Brown WJ, Gebhart SC, Bright S, Carretta E, Ziefle CG, Panjehpour M, Galanko J *et al*: Detection of dysplasia in barrett's esophagus with in vivo depth-resolved nuclear morphology measurements. *Gastroenterology* 2011, 140(1):42-50.

[156] Kelloff GJ, Sigman CC: Assessing intraepithelial neoplasia and drug safety in cancer-preventive drug development. *Nat Rev Cancer* 2007, 7(7):508-518.

[157] Backman V, Wallace MB, Perelman LT, Arendt JT, Gurjar R, Muller MG, Zhang Q, Zonios G, Kline E, McGilligan JA *et al*: Detection of preinvasive cancer cells. *Nature* 2000, 406(6791):35-36.

[158] Weissleder R, Pittet MJ: Imaging in the era of molecular oncology. *Nature* 2008, 452(7187):580-589.

[159] Francisco AL, Correr WR, Pinto CA, Filho JG, Chulam TC, Kurachi C, Kowalski LP: Analysis of surgical margins in oral cancer using in situ fluorescence spectroscopy. *Oral Oncol* 2014.

[160] Bydlon TM, Barry WT, Kennedy SA, Brown JQ, Gallagher JE, Wilke LG, Geradts J, Ramanujam N: Advancing optical imaging for breast margin assessment: an analysis of excisional time, cautery, and patent blue dye on underlying sources of contrast. *PLoS One* 2012, 7(12):e51418.

[161] Pleijhuis R, Timmermans A, De Jong J, De Boer E, Ntziachristos V, Van Dam G: Tissue-simulating Phantoms for Assessing Potential Near-infrared Fluorescence Imaging Applications in Breast Cancer Surgery. *J Vis Exp* 2014(91).

[162] Keereweer S, Sterenborg HJ, Kerrebijn JD, Van Driel PB, Baatenburg de Jong RJ, Lowik CW: Image-guided surgery in head and neck cancer: current practice and future directions of optical imaging. *Head Neck* 2012, 34(1):120-126.

[163] Lane P, Follen M, MacAulay C: Has fluorescence spectroscopy come of age? a case series of oral precancers and cancers using white light, fluorescent light at 405 nm, and reflected light at 545 nm using the Trimira identafi 3000. *Gend Med* 2012, 9(1 SUPPL.):S25-S35.

[164] Lane P, Lam S, Follen M, MacAulay C: Oral fluorescence imaging using 405-nm excitation, aiding the discrimination of cancers and precancers by identifying changes in collagen and elastic breakdown and neovascularization in the underlying stroma. *Gend Med* 2012, 9(1 SUPPL.):S78-S82.e78.

[165] Olivo M, Bhuvaneswari R, Keogh I: Advances in bio-optical imaging for the diagnosis of early oral cancer. *Pharmaceutics* 2011, 3(3):354-378.

[166] Ragazzi M, Piana S, Longo C, Castagnetti F, Foroni M, Ferrari G, Gardini G, Pellacani G: Fluorescence confocal microscopy for pathologists. *Mod Pathol* 2014, 27(3):460-471.

[167] Miyamoto S, Sperry S, Yamashita T, Reddy NP, O'Malley BW, Jr., Li D: Molecular imaging assisted surgery improves survival in a murine head and neck cancer model. *Int J Cancer* 2012, 131(5):1235-1242.

[168] Richards-Kortum R, Sevick-Muraca E: Quantitative optical spectroscopy for tissue diagnosis. *Annu Rev Phys Chem* 1996, 47:555-606.

[169] Pavlova I, Williams M, El-Naggar A, Richards-Kortum R, Gillenwater A: Understanding the biological basis of autofluorescence imaging for oral cancer detection: High-resolution fluorescence microscopy in viable tissue. *Clin Cancer Res* 2008, 14(8): 2396-2404.

[170] Rethman MP, Carpenter W, Cohen EEW, Epstein J, Evans CA, Flalfz CM, Graham FJ, Hujoel PP, Kalmar JR, Koch WM *et al*: Evidence-based clinical recommendations regarding screening for oral squamous cell carcinomas. *J Am Dent Assoc* 2010, 141(5): 509-520.

[171] Poh CF, MacAulay CE, Zhang L, Rosin MP: Tracing the "at-risk" oral mucosa field with autofluorescence: Steps toward clinical impact. *Cancer Prev Res (Phila)* 2009, 2(5): 401-404.

[172] De Veld DCG, Witjes MJH, Sterenborg HJCM, Roodenburg JLN: The status of in vivo autofluorescence spectroscopy and imaging for oral oncology. *Oral Oncol* 2005, 41(2): 117-131.

[173] Roblyer D, Kurachi C, Stepanek V, Williams MD, El-Naggar AK, Lee JJ, Gillenwater AM, Richards-Kortum R: Objective detection and delineation of oral neoplasia using autofluorescence imaging. *Cancer Prev Res (Phila)* 2009, 2(5):423-431.

[174] Pavlova I, Weber CR, Schwarz RA, Williams MD, Gillenwater AM, Richards-Kortum R: Fluorescence spectroscopy of oral tissue: Monte Carlo modeling with site-specific tissue properties. *J Biomed Opt* 2009, 14(1):014009.

[175] Kois JC, Truelove E: Detecting oral cancer: A new technique and case reports. *Dent Today* 2006, 25(10):94-97.

[176] Farah CS, McIntosh L, Georgiou A, McCullough MJ: Efficacy of tissue autofluorescence imaging (VELScope) in the visualization of oral mucosal lesions. *Head Neck* 2012, 34(6):856-862.

[177] Bhatia N, Matias MA, Farah CS: Assessment of a decision making protocol to improve the efficacy of VELscope in general dental practice: A prospective evaluation. *Oral Oncol* 2014.

[178] McIntosh L, McCullough MJ, Farah CS: The assessment of diffused light illumination and acetic acid rinse (Microlux/DL) in the visualisation of oral mucosal lesions. *Oral Oncol* 2009, 45(12):e227-231.

[179] Pazouki S, Chisholm DM, Adi MM, Carmichael G, Farquharson M, Ogden GR, Schor SL, Schor AM: The association between tumour progression and vascularity in the oral mucosa. *J Pathol* 1997, 183(1):39-43.

[180] Raica M, Cimpean AM, Ribatti D: Angiogenesis in pre-malignant conditions. *Eur J Cancer* 2009, 45(11):1924-1934.

[181] Shetty DC, Ahuja P, Taneja DK, Singh Rathore A, Chhina S, Ahuja US, Kumar K, Ahuja A, Rastogi P: Relevance of tumor angiogenesis patterns as a diagnostic value and prognostic indicator in oral precancer and cancer. *Vascular Health and Risk Management* 2011, 7(1):41-47.

[182] Wong Kee Song LM, Adler DG, Conway JD, Diehl DL, Farraye FA, Kantsevoy SV, Kwon R, Mamula P, Rodriguez B, Shah RJ *et al*: Narrow band imaging and multiband imaging. *Gastrointest Endosc* 2008, 67(4):581-589.

[183] Gono K, Yamazaki K, Doguchi N, Nonami T, Obi T, Yamaguchi M, Ohyama N, Machida H, Sano Y, Yoshida S *et al*: Endoscopic observation of tissue by narrowband illumination. *Opt Rev* 2003, 10(4):211-215.

[184] Takano JH, Yakushiji T, Kamiyama I, Nomura T, Katakura A, Takano N, Shibahara T: Detecting early oral cancer: narrowband imaging system observation of the oral mucosa microvasculature. *International journal of oral and maxillofacial surgery* 2010, 39(3):208-213.

[185] Tan NC, Herd MK, Brennan PA, Puxeddu R: The role of narrow band imaging in early detection of head and neck cancer. *Br J Oral Maxillofac Surg* 2012, 50(2):132-136.

[186] Fujii S, Yamazaki M, Muto M, Ochiai A: Microvascular irregularities are associated with composition of squamous epithelial lesions and correlate with subepithelial invasion of superficial-type pharyngeal squamous cell carcinoma. *Histopathology* 2010, 56(4):510-522.

[187] Katada C, Nakayama M, Tanabe S, Naruke A, Koizumi W, Masaki T, Okamoto M, Saigenji K: Narrow band imaging for detecting superficial oral squamous cell carcinoma: a report of two cases. *Laryngoscope* 2007, 117(9):1596-1599.

[188] Tan NCW, Mellor T, Brennan PA, Puxeddu R: Use of narrow band imaging guidance in the management of oral erythroplakia. *Br J Oral Maxillofac Surg* 2011, 49(6):488-490.

[189] Yang SW, Lee YS, Chang LC, Chien HP, Chen TA: Clinical appraisal of endoscopy with narrow-band imaging system in the evaluation and management of homogeneous oral leukoplakia. *ORL J Otorhinolaryngol Relat Spec* 2012, 74(2):102-109.

[190] Gono K, Obi T, Yamaguchi M, Ohyama N, Machida H, Sano Y, Yoshida S, Hamamoto Y, Endo T: Appearance of enhanced tissue features in narrow-band endoscopic imaging. *J Biomed Opt* 2004, 9(3):568-577.

[191] Muto M, Nakane M, Katada C, Sano Y, Ohtsu A, Esumi H, Ebihara S, Yoshida S: Squamous cell carcinoma in situ at oropharyngeal and hypopharyngeal mucosal sites. *Cancer* 2004, 101(6):1375-1381.

[192] Muto M, Katada C, Sano Y, Yoshida S: Narrow band imaging: A new diagnostic approach to visualize angiogenesis in superficial neoplasia. *Clinical Gastroenterology and Hepatology* 2005, 3(7 SUPPL.):S16-S20.

[193] Yoshida T, Inoue H, Usui S, Satodate H, Fukami N, Kudo SE: Narrow-band imaging system with magnifying endoscopy for superficial esophageal lesions. *Gastrointest Endosc* 2004, 59(2):288-295.

[194] Matsumura M, Uedo N, Ishihara R, Iishi H, Fujii T, Tomita Y: A case of intraepithelial neoplasia in the oropharynx detected by endoscopic screening with narrow-band imaging videoendoscopy. *Gastrointest Endosc* 2008, 68(1):146-147.

[195] Lin YC, Wang WH: Narrow-band imaging for detecting early recurrent nasopharyngeal carcinoma. *Head Neck* 2011, 33(4):591-594.

[196] Piazza C: Is narrow band imaging the ideal screening tool for mucosal head and neck cancer? *Oral Oncol* 2011, 47(5):313.

[197] Orita Y, Kawabata K, Mitani H, Fukushima H, Tanaka S, Yoshimoto S, Yamamoto N: Can narrow-band imaging be used to determine the surgical margin of superficial hypopharyngeal cancer? *Acta medica Okayama* 2008, 62(3):205-208.

[198] Watanabe A, Taniguchi M, Tsujie H, Hosokawa M, Fujita M, Sasaki S: The value of narrow band imaging for early detection of laryngeal cancer. *European Archives of Oto-Rhino-Laryngology* 2009, 266(7):1017-1023.

[199] Watanabe A, Taniguchi M, Tsujie H, Hosokawa M, Fujita M, Sasaki S: The value of narrow band imaging endoscope for early head and neck cancer. *Otolaryngology-Head and Neck Surgery* 2008, 138(4):446-451.

[200] Igarashi Y, Okano N, Ito K, Suzuki T, Mimura T: Effectiveness of peroral cholangioscopy and narrow band imaging for endoscopically diagnosing the bile duct cancer. *Dig Endosc* 2009, 21 Suppl 1:S101-102.

[201] Itoi T, Sofuni A, Itokawa F, Tsuchiya T, Kurihara T: Evaluation of peroral videocholangioscopy using narrow-band imaging for diagnosis of intraductal papillary neoplasm of the bile duct. *Dig Endosc* 2009, 21 Suppl 1:S103-107.

[202] Itoi T, Tsuji S, Sofuni A, Itokawa F, Kurihara T, Tsuchiya T, Ishii K, Ikeuchi N, Igarashi M, Gotoda T *et al*: A novel approach emphasizing preoperative margin enhancement of tumor of the major duodenal papilla with narrow-band imaging in comparison to indigo carmine chromoendoscopy (with videos). *Gastrointest Endosc* 2009, 69(1):136-141.

[203] Kiyotoki S, Nishikawa J, Satake M, Fukagawa Y, Shirai Y, Hamabe K, Saito M, Okamoto T, Sakaida I: Usefulness of magnifying endoscopy with narrow-band imaging for determining gastric tumor margin. *J Gastroenterol Hepatol* 2010, 25(10):1636-1641.

[204] Nagahama T, Yao K, Maki S, Yasaka M, Takaki Y, Matsui T, Tanabe H, Iwashita A, Ota A: Usefulness of magnifying endoscopy with narrow-band imaging for determining the horizontal extent of early gastric cancer when there is an unclear margin by chromoendoscopy (with video). *Gastrointest Endosc* 2011, 74(6):1259-1267.

[205] Muto M, Horimatsu T, Ezoe Y, Morita S, Miyamoto S: Improving visualization techniques by narrow band imaging and magnification endoscopy. *Journal of Gastroenterology and Hepatology (Australia)* 2009, 24(8):1333-1346.

[206] Piazza C, Dessouky O, Peretti G, Cocco D, De Benedetto L, Nicolai P: Narrow-band imaging: a new tool for evaluation of head and neck squamous cell carcinomas. Review of the literature. *Acta otorhinolaryngologica Italica : organo ufficiale della Societa italiana di otorinolaringologia e chirurgia cervico-facciale* 2008, 28(2):49-54.

[207] Muto M, Minashi K, Yano T, Saito Y, Oda I, Nonaka S, Omori T, Sugiura H, Goda K, Kaise M *et al*: Early Detection of Superficial Squamous Cell Carcinoma in the Head and Neck Region and Esophagus by Narrow Band Imaging: A Multicenter Randomized Controlled Trial. *Journal of Clinical Oncology* 2010, 28(9):1566-1572.

[208] Piazza C, Cocco D, Del Bon F, Mangili S, Nicolai P, Majorana A, Bolzoni Villaret A, Peretti G: Narrow band imaging and high definition television in evaluation of oral

and oropharyngeal squamous cell cancer: a prospective study. *Oral Oncol* 2010, 46(4): 307-310.

[209] Piazza C, Cocco D, Del Bon F, Mangili S, Nicolai P, Peretti G: Narrow band imaging and high definition television in the endoscopic evaluation of upper aero-digestive tract cancer. *Acta otorhinolaryngologica Italica : organo ufficiale della Societa italiana di otorinolaringologia e chirurgia cervico-facciale* 2011, 31(2):70-75.

[210] Fielding D, Agnew J, Wright D, Hodge R: Autofluorescence improves pretreatment mucosal assessment in head and neck cancer patients. *Otolaryngol Head Neck Surg* 2010, 142(3):S20-S26.

[211] Nguyen P, Bashirzadeh F, Hodge R, Agnew J, Farah CS, Duhig E, Clarke B, Perry-Keene J, Botros D, Masters IB *et al*: High specificity of combined narrow band imaging and autofluorescence mucosal assessment of patients with head and neck cancer. *Head Neck* 2013, 35(5):619-625.

[212] Vu AN, Farah CS: Efficacy of narrow band imaging for detection and surveillance of potentially malignant and malignant lesions in the oral cavity and oropharynx: A systematic review. *Oral Oncol* 2014.

[213] Yang SW, Lee YS, Chang LC, Chien HP, Chen TA: Light sources used in evaluating oral leukoplakia: broadband white light versus narrowband imaging. *International journal of oral and maxillofacial surgery* 2013, 42(6):693-701.

[214] Roblyer D, Richards-Kortum R, Sokolov K, El-Naggar AK, Williams MD, Kurachi C, Gillenwater AM: Multispectral optical imaging device for in vivo detection of oral neoplasia. *J Biomed Opt* 2008, 13(2):024019.

[215] Chi C, Du Y, Ye J, Kou D, Qiu J, Wang J, Tian J, Chen X: Intraoperative imaging-guided cancer surgery: from current fluorescence molecular imaging methods to future multi-modality imaging technology. *Theranostics* 2014, 4(11):1072-1084.

[216] Dammann F, Bootz F, Cohnen M, Hassfeld S, Tatagiba M, Kosling S: Diagnostic imaging modalities in head and neck disease. *Deutsches Arzteblatt international* 2014, 111(23-24):417-423.

[217] Shah AT, Demory Beckler M, Walsh AJ, Jones WP, Pohlmann PR, Skala MC: Optical metabolic imaging of treatment response in human head and neck squamous cell carcinoma. *PLoS One* 2014, 9(3):e90746.

[218] Nguyen QT, Tsien RY: Fluorescence-guided surgery with live molecular navigation--a new cutting edge. *Nat Rev Cancer* 2013, 13(9):653-662.

[219] Kircher MF, Willmann JK: Molecular body imaging: MR imaging, CT, and US. Part I. Principles. *Radiology* 2012, 263(3):633-643.

[220] Elias DR, Thorek DLJ, Chen AK, Czupryna J, Tsourkas A: In vivo imaging of cancer biomarkers using activatable molecular probes. *Cancer Biomarkers* 2008, 4(6):287-305.

[221] Vogelstein B, Kinzler KW: Cancer genes and the pathways they control. *Nature Medicine* 2004, 10(8):789-799.

[222] Hoeben BA, Bussink J, Troost EG, Oyen WJ, Kaanders JH: Molecular PET imaging for biology-guided adaptive radiotherapy of head and neck cancer. *Acta oncologica (Stockholm, Sweden)* 2013, 52(7):1257-1271.

[223] Hoeben BA, Starmans MH, Leijenaar RT, Dubois LJ, van der Kogel AJ, Kaanders JH, Boutros PC, Lambin P, Bussink J: Systematic analysis of 18F-FDG PET and metabolism, proliferation and hypoxia markers for classification of head and neck tumors. *BMC cancer* 2014, 14:130.

[224] Loja MN, Luo Z, Greg Farwell D, Luu QC, Donald PJ, Amott D, Truong AQ, Gandour-Edwards RF, Nitin N: Optical molecular imaging detects changes in extracellular pH with the development of head and neck cancer. *Int J Cancer* 2013, 132(7): 1613-1623.

[225] Bakker Schut TC, Witjes MJ, Sterenborg HJ, Speelman OC, Roodenburg JL, Marple ET, Bruining HA, Puppels GJ: In vivo detection of dysplastic tissue by Raman spectroscopy. *Anal Chem* 2000, 72(24):6010-6018.

[226] Kendall C, Stone N, Shepherd N, Geboes K, Warren B, Bennett R, Barr H: Raman spectroscopy, a potential tool for the objective identification and classification of neoplasia in Barrett's oesophagus. *J Pathol* 2003, 200(5):602-609.

[227] Shim MG, Song LM, Marcon NE, Wilson BC: In vivo near-infrared Raman spectroscopy: demonstration of feasibility during clinical gastrointestinal endoscopy. *Photochem Photobiol* 2000, 72(1):146-150.

[228] Molckovsky A, Song LM, Shim MG, Marcon NE, Wilson BC: Diagnostic potential of near-infrared Raman spectroscopy in the colon: differentiating adenomatous from hyperplastic polyps. *Gastrointest Endosc* 2003, 57(3):396-402.

[229] Haka AS, Volynskaya Z, Gardecki JA, Nazemi J, Lyons J, Hicks D, Fitzmaurice M, Dasari RR, Crowe JP, Feld MS: In vivo margin assessment during partial mastectomy breast surgery using raman spectroscopy. *Cancer Res* 2006, 66(6):3317-3322.

[230] Stone N, Stavroulaki P, Kendall C, Birchall M, Barr H: Raman spectroscopy for early detection of laryngeal malignancy: preliminary results. *Laryngoscope* 2000, 110(10 Pt 1):1756-1763.

[231] Lau DP, Huang Z, Lui H, Anderson DW, Berean K, Morrison MD, Shen L, Zeng H: Raman spectroscopy for optical diagnosis in the larynx: preliminary findings. *Lasers Surg Med* 2005, 37(3):192-200.

[232] Keller MD, Wilson RH, Mycek MA, Mahadevan-Jansen A: Monte Carlo model of spatially offset Raman spectroscopy for breast tumor margin analysis. *Appl Spectrosc* 2010, 64(6):607-614.

[233] Ellis DI, Cowcher DP, Ashton L, O'Hagan S, Goodacre R: Illuminating disease and enlightening biomedicine: Raman spectroscopy as a diagnostic tool. *Analyst* 2013, 138(14):3871-3884.

[234] Tollefson M, Magera J, Sebo T, Cohen J, Drauch A, Maier J, Frank I: Raman spectral imaging of prostate cancer: can Raman molecular imaging be used to augment standard histopathology? *BJU Int* 2010, 106(4):484-488.

[235] Crow P, Uff JS, Farmer JA, Wright MP, Stone N: The use of Raman spectroscopy to identify and characterize transitional cell carcinoma in vitro. *BJU Int* 2004, 93(9): 1232-1236.

[236] Johnson JT, Branstetter BF: PET/CT in head and neck oncology: State-of-the-art 2013. *Laryngoscope* 2014, 124(4):913-915.

[237] Partovi S, Kohan A, Rubbert C, Vercher-Conejero JL, Gaeta C, Yuh R, Zipp L, Herrmann KA, Robbin MR, Lee Z *et al*: Clinical oncologic applications of PET/MRI: a new horizon. *American journal of nuclear medicine and molecular imaging* 2014, 4(2):202-212.

[238] Al-Nabhani KZ, Syed R, Michopoulou S, Alkalbani J, Afaq A, Panagiotidis E, O'Meara C, Groves A, Ell P, Bomanji J: Qualitative and quantitative comparison of PET/CT and PET/MR imaging in clinical practice. *J Nucl Med* 2014, 55(1):88-94.

[239] Kubiessa K, Purz S, Gawlitza M, Kuhn A, Fuchs J, Steinhoff KG, Boehm A, Sabri O, Kluge R, Kahn T *et al*: Initial clinical results of simultaneous F-18-FDG PET/MRI in comparison to F-18-FDG PET/CT in patients with head and neck cancer. *Eur J Nucl Med Mol Imaging* 2014, 41(4):639-648.

[240] Kuhn FP, Hullner M, Mader CE, Kastrinidis N, Huber GF, von Schulthess GK, Kollias S, Veit-Haibach P: Contrast-enhanced PET/MR imaging versus contrast-enhanced PET/CT in head and neck cancer: how much MR information is needed? *J Nucl Med* 2014, 55(4):551-558.

[241] Partovi S, Kohan A, Vercher-Conejero JL, Rubbert C, Margevicius S, Schluchter MD, Gaeta C, Faulhaber P, Robbin MR: Qualitative and quantitative performance of 18F-FDG-PET/MRI versus 18F-FDG-PET/CT in patients with head and neck cancer. *AJNR American journal of neuroradiology* 2014.

[242] Queiroz M, Hullner M, Kuhn F, Huber G, Meerwein C, Kollias S, von Schulthess G, Veit-Haibach P: PET/MRI and PET/CT in follow-up of head and neck cancer patients. *Eur J Nucl Med Mol Imaging* 2014, 41(6):1066-1075.

[243] Varoquaux A, Rager O, Poncet A, Delattre BMA, Ratib O, Becker CD, Dulguerov P, Dulguerov N, Zaidi H, Becker M: Detection and quantification of focal uptake in head and neck tumours: F-18-FDG PET/MR versus PET/CT. *Eur J Nucl Med Mol Imaging* 2014, 41(3):462-475.

[244] Kanda T, Kitajima K, Suenaga Y, Konishi J, Sasaki R, Morimoto K, Saito M, Otsuki N, Nibu K, Sugimura K: Value of retrospective image fusion of F-18-FDG PET and MRI

for preoperative staging of head and neck cancer: Comparison with PET/CT and contrast-enhanced neck MRI. *Eur J Radiol* 2013, 82(11):2005-2010.

[245] Lee G, I H, Kim SJ, Jeong YJ, Kim IJ, Pak K, Park DY, Kim GH: Clinical Implication of PET/MR Imaging in Preoperative Esophageal Cancer Staging: Comparison with PET/CT, Endoscopic Ultrasonography, and CT. *J Nucl Med* 2014.

[246] Evangelista L, Cervino AR, Chondrogiannis S, Marzola MC, Maffione AM, Colletti PM, Muzzio PC, Rubello D: Comparison between anatomical cross-sectional imaging and F-18-FDG PET/CT in the staging, restaging, treatment response, and long-term surveillance of squamous cell head and neck cancer: a systematic literature overview. *Nucl Med Commun* 2014, 35(2):123-134.

[247] Arias F, Chicata V, Garcia-Velloso MJ, Asin G, Uzcanga M, Eito C, Quilez I, Viudez A, Saenz J, Hernandez I *et al*: Impact of initial FDG PET/CT in the management plan of patients with locally advanced head and neck cancer. *Clinical & translational oncology : official publication of the Federation of Spanish Oncology Societies and of the National Cancer Institute of Mexico* 2014.

[248] Adkins D, Ley J, Dehdashti F, Siegel MJ, Wildes TM, Michel L, Trinkaus K, Siegel BA: A prospective trial comparing FDG-PET/CT and CT to assess tumor response to cetuximab in patients with incurable squamous cell carcinoma of the head and neck. *Cancer medicine* 2014.

[249] Garcheva M, Zlatareva D, Gocheva L: Positron emission tomography combined with computed tomography for diagnosis of synchronous tumors. *Klinicka onkologie : casopis Ceske a Slovenske onkologicke spolecnosti* 2014, 27(4):283-286.

[250] Bhatnagar P, Subesinghe M, Patel C, Prestwich R, Scarsbrook AF: Functional imaging for radiation treatment planning, response assessment, and adaptive therapy in head and neck cancer. *Radiographics : a review publication of the Radiological Society of North America, Inc* 2013, 33(7):1909-1929.

[251] Bussink J, van Herpen CML, Kaanders JHAM, Oyen WJG: PET-CT for response assessment and treatment adaptation in head and neck cancer. *Lancet Oncol* 2010, 11(7): 661-669.

[252] Nordsmark M, Bentzen SM, Rudat V, Brizel D, Lartigau E, Stadler P, Becker A, Adam M, Molls M, Dunst J *et al*: Prognostic value of tumor oxygenation in 397 head and neck tumors after primary radiation therapy. An international multi-center study. *Radiother Oncol* 2005, 77(1):18-24.

[253] Eschmann SM, Paulsen F, Reimold M, Dittmann H, Welz S, Reischl G, Machulla HJ, Bares R: Prognostic impact of hypoxia imaging with F-18-misonidazole PET in non-small cell lung cancer and head and neck cancer before radiotherapy. *J Nucl Med* 2005, 46(2):253-260.

[254] Rischin D, Hicks RJ, Fisher R, Binns D, Corry J, Porceddu S, Peters LJ: Prognostic significance of [F-18]-misonidazole positron emission tomography-detected tumor hy-

poxia in patients with advanced head and neck cancer randomly assigned to chemoradiation with or without tirapazamine: A substudy of Trans-Tasman Radiation Oncology Group study 98.02. *J Clin Oncol* 2006, 24(13):2098-2104.

[255] Thorwarth D, Eschmann S-M, Holzner F, Paulsen F, Alber M: Combined uptake of [(18)F]FDG and [(18)F]FMISO correlates with radiation therapy outcome in head-and-neck cancer patients. *Radiother Oncol* 2006, 80(2):151-156.

[256] Zimny M, Gagel B, DiMartino E, Hamacher K, Coenen HH, Westhofen M, Eble M, Buell U, Reinartz P: FDG - a marker of tumour hypoxia? A comparison with [F-18] fluoromisonidazole and pO(2)-polarography in metastatic head and neck cancer. *Eur J Nucl Med Mol Imaging* 2006, 33(12):1426-1431.

[257] Hendrickson K, Phillips M, Smith W, Peterson L, Krohn K, Rajendran J: Hypoxia imaging with [F-18] FMISO-PET in head and neck cancer: Potential for guiding intensity modulated radiation therapy in overcoming hypoxia-induced treatment resistance. *Radiother Oncol* 2011, 101(3):369-375.

[258] Lee NY, Mechalakos JG, Nehmeh S, Lin Z, Squire OD, Cai S, Chan K, Zanzonico PB, Greco C, Ling CC *et al*: Fluorine-18-labeled fluoromisonidazole positron emission and computed tomography-guided intensity-modulated radiotherapy for head and neck cancer: A feasibility study. *Int J Radiat Oncol Biol Phys* 2008, 70(1):2-13.

[259] Rajendran JG, Hendrickson KRG, Spence AM, Muzi M, Krohn KA, Mankoff DA: Hypoxia imaging-directed radiation treatment planning. *Eur J Nucl Med Mol Imaging* 2006, 33 Suppl 1:44-53.

[260] Thorwarth D, Eschmann S-M, Paulsen F, Alber M: Hypoxia dose painting by numbers: A planning study. *Int J Radiat Oncol Biol Phys* 2007, 68(1):291-300.

[261] Nehmeh SA, Lee NY, Schroder H, Squire O, Zanzonico PB, Erdi YE, Greco C, Mageras G, Pham HS, Larson SM *et al*: Reproducibility of intratumor distribution of F-18-fluoromisonidazole in head and neck cancer. *Int J Radiat Oncol Biol Phys* 2008, 70(1): 235-242.

[262] Lin Z, Mechalakos J, Nehmeh S, Schoder H, Lee N, Humm J, Ling CC: The influence of changes in tumor hypoxia on dose-painting treatment plans based on (18)F-FMISO positron emission tomography. *Int J Radiat Oncol Biol Phys* 2008, 70(4):1219-1228.

[263] Wang W, Lee NY, Georgi J-C, Narayanan M, Guillem J, Schoeder H, Humm JL: Pharmacokinetic analysis of hypoxia F-18-fluoromisonidazole dynamic PET in head and neck cancer. *J Nucl Med* 2010, 51(1):37-45.

[264] Piert M, Machulla HJ, Picchio M, Reischl G, Ziegler S, Kumar P, Wester HJ, Beck R, McEwan AJB, Wiebe LI *et al*: Hypoxia-specific tumor imaging with F-18-fluoroazomycin arabinoside. *J Nucl Med* 2005, 46(1):106-113.

[265] Gronroos T, Eskola I, Lehtio K, Minn H, Marjamaki P, Bergman J, Haaparanta M, Forsback S, Solin O: Pharmacokinetics of [F-18]FETNIM: A potential hypoxia marker for PET. *J Nucl Med* 2001, 42(9):1397-1404.

[266] Vavere AL, Lewis JS: Cu-ATSM: A radiopharmaceutical for the PET imaging of hypoxia. *Dalton Trans* 2007(43):4893-4902.

[267] Minagawa Y, Shizukuishi K, Koike I, Horiuchi C, Watanuki K, Hata M, Omura M, Odagiri K, Tohnai I, Inoue T *et al*: Assessment of tumor hypoxia by Cu-62-ATSM PET/CT as a predictor of response in head and neck cancer: a pilot study. *Ann Nucl Med* 2011, 25(5):339-345.

[268] Chao KSC, Bosch WR, Mutic S, Lewis JS, Dehdashti F, Mintun MA, Dempsey JF, Perez CA, Purdy JA, Welch MJ: A novel approach to overcome hypoxic tumor resistance: Cu-ATSM-guided intensity-modulated radiation therapy. *Int J Radiat Oncol Biol Phys* 2001, 49(4):1171-1182.

[269] Weber WA: Monitoring tumor response to therapy with F-18-FLT PET. *J Nucl Med* 2010, 51(6):841-844.

[270] Rasey JS, Grierson JR, Wiens LW, Kolb PD, Schwartz JL: Validation of FLT uptake as a measure of thymidine kinase-1 activity in A549 carcinoma cells. *J Nucl Med* 2002, 43(9):1210-1217.

[271] Troost EGC, Bussink J, Hoffmann AL, Boerman OC, Oyen WJG, Kaanders JHAM: F-18-FLT PET/CT for early response monitoring and dose escalation in oropharyngeal tumors. *J Nucl Med* 2010, 51(6):866-874.

[272] Troost EGC, Vogel WV, Merkx MAW, Slootweg PJ, Marres HAM, Peeters WJM, Bussink J, van der Kogel AJ, Oyen WJG, Kaanders JHAM: F-18-FLT PET does not discriminate between reactive and metastatic lymph nodes in primary head and neck cancer patients. *J Nucl Med* 2007, 48(5):726-735.

[273] Cotter TG: Apoptosis and cancer: the genesis of a research field. *Nat Rev Cancer* 2009, 9(7):501-507.

[274] Hoebers FJP, Kartachova M, de Bois J, van den Brekel MWM, van Tinteren H, van Herk M, Rasch CRN, Olmos RAV, Verheij M: Tc-99m Hynic-rh-Annexin V scintigraphy for in vivo imaging of apoptosis in patients with head and neck cancer treated with chemoradiotherapy. *Eur J Nucl Med Mol Imaging* 2008, 35(3):509-518.

[275] Hoglund J, Shirvan A, Antoni G, Gustavsson S-A, Langstrom B, Ringheim A, Sorensen J, Ben-Ami M, Ziv I: F-18-ML-10, a PET tracer for apoptosis: first human study. *J Nucl Med* 2011, 52(5):720-725.

[276] Hoffman RM: Altered methionine metabolism, DNA methylation and oncogene expression in carcinogenesis. A review and synthesis. *Biochim Biophys Acta* 1984, 738(1-2):49-87.

[277] Leskinenkallio S, Nagren K, Lehikoinen P, Ruotsalainen U, Teras M, Joensuu H: Carbon-11-methionine and PET is an effective method to image head and neck cancer. *J Nucl Med* 1992, 33(5):691-695.

[278] Lindholm P, Leskinenkallio S, Minn H, Bergman J, Haaparanta M, Lehikoinen P, Nagren K, Ruotsalainen U, Teras M, Joensuu H: Comparison of fluorine-18-fluorodeoxyglucose and carbon-11-methionine in head and neck cancer. *J Nucl Med* 1993, 34(10):1711-1716.

[279] Lindholm P, Leskinenkallio S, Grenman R, Lehikoinen P, Nagren K, Teras M, Ruotsalainen U, Joensuu H: Evaluation of response to radiotherapy in dead-end neck-cancer by positron emission tomography and [C-11] methionine. *Int J Radiat Oncol Biol Phys* 1995, 32(3):787-794.

[280] Chesnay E, Babin E, Constans JM, Agostini D, Bequignon A, Regeasse A, Sobrio F, Moreau S: Early response to chemotherapy in hypopharyngeal cancer: Assessment with C-11-methionine PET, correlation with morphologic response, and clinical outcome. *J Nucl Med* 2003, 44(4):526-532.

[281] Nuutinen J, Jyrkkio S, Lehikoinen P, Lindholm P, Minn H: Evaluation of early response to radiotherapy in head and neck cancer measured with [C-11]methionine-positron emission tomography. *Radiother Oncol* 1999, 52(3):225-232.

[282] Balogova S, Perie S, Kerrou K, Grahek D, Montravers F, Angelard B, Susini B, El Chater P, St Guily JL, Talbot JN: Prospective comparison of FDG and FET PET/CT in patients with head and neck squamous cell carcinoma. *Mol Imaging Biol* 2008, 10(6): 364-373.

[283] Haerle SK, Fischer DR, Schmid DT, Ahmad N, Huber GF, Buck A: F-18-FET PET/CT in advanced head and neck squamous cell carcinoma: an intra-individual comparison with F-18-FDG PET/CT. *Mol Imaging Biol* 2011, 13(5):1036-1042.

[284] Pauleit D, Zimmermann A, Stoffels G, Bauer D, Risse J, Fluss MO, Hamacher K, Coenen HH, Langen KJ: F-18-FET PET compared with F-18-FDG PET and CT in patients with head and neck cancer. *J Nucl Med* 2006, 47(2):256-261.

[285] Wester HJ, Herz M, Weber W, Heiss P, Senekowitsch-Schmidtke R, Schwaiger M, Stocklin G: Synthesis and radiopharmacology of O-(2-[F-18]fluoroethyl)-L-tyrosine for tumor imaging. *J Nucl Med* 1999, 40(1):205-212.

[286] Roivainen A, Forsback S, Gronroos T, Lehikoinen P, Kahkonen M, Sutinen E, Minn H: Blood metabolism of [methyl-C-11]choline; implications for in vivo imaging with positron emission tomography. *Eur J Nucl Med* 2000, 27(1):25-32.

[287] Khan N, Oriuchi N, Ninomiya H, Higuchi T, Kamada H, Endo K: Positron emission tomographic imaging with C-11-choline in differential diagnosis of head and neck tumors: comparison with F-18-FDG PET. *Ann Nucl Med* 2004, 18(5):409-417.

[288] Ito K, Yokoyama J, Kubota K, Morooka M, Shiibashi M, Matsuda H: F-18-FDG versus C-11-choline PET/CT for the imaging of advanced head and neck cancer after com-

bined intra-arterial chemotherapy and radiotherapy: the time period during which PET/CT can reliably detect non-recurrence. *Eur J Nucl Med Mol Imaging* 2010, 37(7): 1318-1327.

[289] Chen YJ, Wu SC, Chen CY, Tzou SC, Cheng TL, Huang YF, Yuan SS, Wang YM: Peptide-based MRI contrast agent and near-infrared fluorescent probe for intratumoral legumain detection. *Biomaterials* 2014, 35(1):304-315.

[290] Luo T, Huang P, Gao G, Shen G, Fu S, Cui D, Zhou C, Ren Q: Mesoporous silica-coated gold nanorods with embedded indocyanine green for dual mode X-ray CT and NIR fluorescence imaging. *Opt Express* 2011, 19(18):17030-17039.

[291] Peloso A, Franchi E, Canepa MC, Barbieri L, Briani L, Ferrario J, Bianco C, Quaretti P, Brugnatelli S, Dionigi P *et al*: Combined use of intraoperative ultrasound and indocyanine green fluorescence imaging to detect liver metastases from colorectal cancer. *HPB (Oxford)* 2013, 15(12):928-934.

[292] Jin XJ, Zhou L, Zhao AG: Mutants of p53 gene presence in laryngeal carcinoma and adjacent histopathologically normal tissue. *Orl-Journal for Oto-Rhino-Laryngology and Its Related Specialties* 2000, 62(3):140-142.

[293] van der Toorn PPG, Veltman JA, Bot FJ, de Jong JMA, Manni JJ, Ramaekers FCS, Hopman AHN: Mapping of resection margins of oral cancer for p53 overexpression and chromosome instability to detect residual (pre)malignant cells. *J Pathol* 2001, 193(1):66-72.

[294] Shin DM, Charuruks N, Lippman SM, Lee JJ, Ro JY, Hong WK, Hittelman WN: p53 protein accumulation and genomic instability in head and neck multistep tumorigenesis. *Cancer epidemiology, biomarkers & prevention : a publication of the American Association for Cancer Research, cosponsored by the American Society of Preventive Oncology* 2001, 10(6):603-609.

[295] Szukala K, Brieger J, Bruch K, Biczysko W, Wierzbicka M, Szyfter W, Szyfter K: Loss of heterozygosity on chromosome arm 13q in larynx cancer patients: analysis of tumor, margin and clinically unchanged mucosa. *Medical science monitor : international medical journal of experimental and clinical research* 2004, 10(6):Cr233-240.

[296] Shaw RJ, Hall GL, Woolgar JA, Lowe D, Rogers SN, Field JK, Liloglou T, Risk JM: Quantitative methylation analysis of resection margins and lymph nodes in oral squamous cell carcinoma. *Br J Oral Maxillofac Surg* 2007, 45(8):617-622.

[297] Barrera JE, Ai H, Pan ZX, Meyers AD, Varella-Garcia M: Malignancy detection by molecular cytogenetics in clinically normal mucosa adjacent to head and neck tumors. *Arch Otolaryngol Head Neck Surg* 1998, 124(8):847-851.

[298] Voravud N, Shin DM, Ro JY, Lee JS, Hong WK, Hittelman WN: Increased polysomies of chromosome-7 and chromosome-17 during head and neck multistage tumorigenesis. *Cancer Res* 1993, 53(12):2874-2883.

[299] Fabricius EM, Gurr U, Wildner GP: Telomerase activity levels in the surgical margin and tumour distant tissue of the squamous cell carcinoma of the head-and-neck. *Anal Cell Pathol* 2002, 24(1):25-39.

[300] Graveland AP, de Maaker M, Braakhuis BJ, de Bree R, Eerenstein SE, Bloemena E, Leemans CR, Brakenhoff RH: Molecular detection of minimal residual cancer in surgical margins of head and neck cancer patients. *Cell Oncol* 2009, 31(4):317-328.

[301] Dasgupta S, Koch R, Westra WH, Califano JA, Ha PK, Sidransky D, Koch WM: Mitochondrial DNA mutation in normal margins and tumors of recurrent head and neck squamous cell carcinoma patients. *Cancer Prev Res (Phila)* 2010, 3(9):1205-1211.

[302] Huang X, Pateromichelakis S, Hills A, Sherriff M, Lyons A, Langdon J, Odell E, Morgan P, Harrison J, Partridge M: p53 mutations in deep tissues are more strongly associated with recurrence than mutation-positive mucosal margins. *Clin Cancer Res* 2007, 13(20):6099-6106.

[303] Ogbureke KU, Weinberger PM, Looney SW, Li L, Fisher LW: Expressions of matrix metalloproteinase-9 (MMP-9), dentin sialophosphoprotein (DSPP), and osteopontin (OPN) at histologically negative surgical margins may predict recurrence of oral squamous cell carcinoma. *Oncotarget* 2012, 3(3):286-298.

[304] Reis PP, Waldron L, Perez-Ordonez B, Pintilie M, Galloni NN, Xuan Y, Cervigne NK, Warner GC, Makitie AA, Simpson C *et al*: A gene signature in histologically normal surgical margins is predictive of oral carcinoma recurrence. *BMC cancer* 2011, 11:437.

[305] Montebugnoli L, Gissi DB, Badiali G, Marchetti C, Cervellati F, Farnedi A, Foschini MP: Ki-67 from clinically and histologically "normal" distant mucosa as prognostic marker in early-stage (T1-T2N0) oral squamous cell carcinoma: a prospective study. *Journal of oral and maxillofacial surgery : official journal of the American Association of Oral and Maxillofacial Surgeons* 2011, 69(10):2579-2584.

[306] Temam S, Casiraghi O, Lahaye JB, Bosq J, Zhou X, Julieron M, Mamelle G, Lee JJ, Mao L, Luboinski B *et al*: Tetranucleotide microsatellite instability in surgical margins for prediction of local recurrence of head and neck squamous cell carcinoma. *Clin Cancer Res* 2004, 10(12):4022-4028.

[307] Handschel J, Oz D, Pomjanski N, Depprich R, Ommerborn MA, Braunstein S, Kuebler NR, Meyer U, Boecking A: Additional use of DNA-image cytometry improves the assessment of resection margins. J Oral Pathol Med 2007, 36(8):472-475.

[308] Zhao H, Ren J, Zhuo X, Ye H, Zou J, Liu S: Prognostic significance of Survivin and CD44v6 in laryngeal cancer surgical margins. Journal of cancer research and clinical oncology 2008, 134(10):1051-1058.

[309] Schaaij-Visser TB, Graveland AP, Gauci S, Braakhuis BJ, Buijze M, Heck AJ, Kuik DJ, Bloemena E, Leemans CR, Slijper M et al: Differential Proteomics Identifies Protein Biomarkers That Predict Local Relapse of Head and Neck Squamous Cell Carcinomas. Clin Cancer Res 2009, 15(24):7666-7675.

Chapter 5

Oral Squamous Cell Carcinoma in Young Population — Risk Factors, Clinical Presentation, and Prognosis

Ligia Buloto Schmitd, Kellen Cristine Tjioe,
Agnes Assao and Denise Tostes Oliveira

Additional information is available at the end of the chapter

http://dx.doi.org/10.5772/60712

1. Introduction

The oral squamous cell carcinoma is a particular type of cancer classically described as a tobacco- and alcohol-related disease affecting mostly elderly male patients. However, epidemiologic studies have demonstrated an increasing incidence of young individuals with oral cancer. Interestingly, the clinicopathological profile, etiology, risk factors, and outcome of patients with early-onset disease seem to present several differences compared to late-onset oral carcinoma and these discrepancies are discussed below.

2. Clinical manifestations

Retrospective studies including elderly and young patients have shown that the incidence of squamous cell carcinoma (SCC) of the mouth in young people is low but presents an increasing tendency [1]. In fact, there is certain heterogeneity of the cutoff age employed in the studies. Most authors consider young patients as those who are under 40 or 45 years [2-6] whereas few investigations select individuals under 20 or 30 years [7-9]. The incidence of oral cancer in patients younger than 40 years of age varies between 0.4–3.6%, but it can reach 6.7% in studies considering 45 years as the cutoff point [10]. Due to its rarity, most investigations deal with a small sample of patients, and conflicting results have been published regarding the epidemiological aspects of oral SCC.

The clear male predominance found in late-onset lesions is not found in the early-onset counterparts. Men are still more affected than women but only slightly more, with a F:M ratio varying from 1:1.2 to 1:4.9 [11, 12]. These data show an evident augmentation in the number of young women affected by oral SCC. The differences between sex distribution previously observed may be due to smoking and drinking habits, which are more socially acceptable for both genders currently [10].

The most common oral subsite for SCC in young patients is the tongue, with 39–77% of the cases [13, 14]. A study conducted in Taiwan found a higher incidence of oral SCC in the buccal area (53.6%) in comparison with the tongue (42, 8%), but betel chewing was common among these patients [15]. Other retrospective reports in Germany and Brazil showed a slightly higher incidence of oral SCC in the floor of the mouth, followed by the mobile tongue [12, 16].

The typical clinical appearance of oral SCC in young patients is an ulcer, often intermixed with white plaque and/or reddish areas. Kuriakose *et al.* [17] noted that lesions in young patients were predominantly invasive as compared with the exophytic lesions found in older patients [10, 17]. On the other hand, Falaki *et al.* [18] reported exophytic lesion with ulcer as the most common clinical presentation in younger individuals.

Figures 1 and 2 illustrate a 35-year-old young man who presented with a white plaque intermixed with erythroplastic areas in the right border of the tongue. The duration of the lesion was of one year, and the patient reported slight pain. Moreover, the individual did neither consume tobacco nor alcohol. Incisional biopsy confirmed the diagnosis of SCC that was staged lately as T2N0M0. The patient was submitted to partial glossectomy with supra-omohyoid selective neck dissection of the same side and radiotherapy. The one-year follow-up was uneventful.

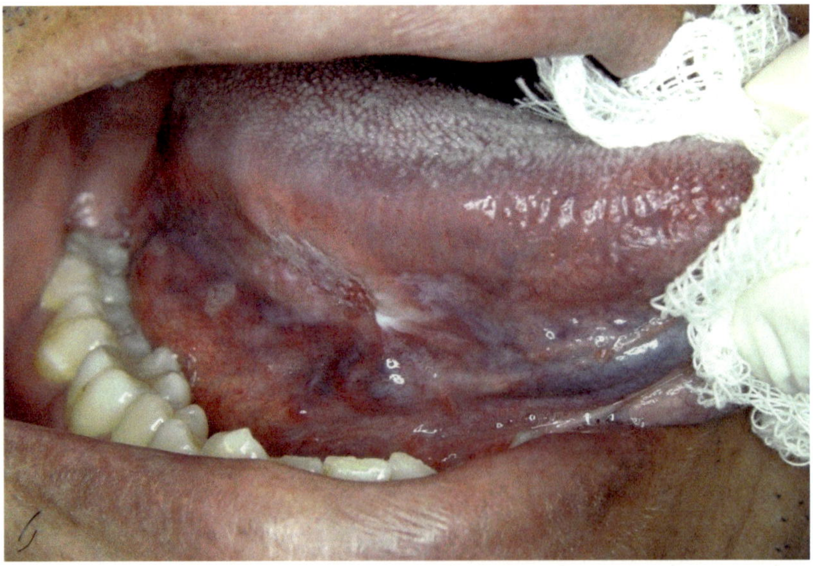

Figure 1. Clinical features of oral SCC in young patient – presence of white plaque and ulceration at the right lateral surface of the mobile tongue of a 35-year-old patient.

http://dx.doi.org/10.5772/60712

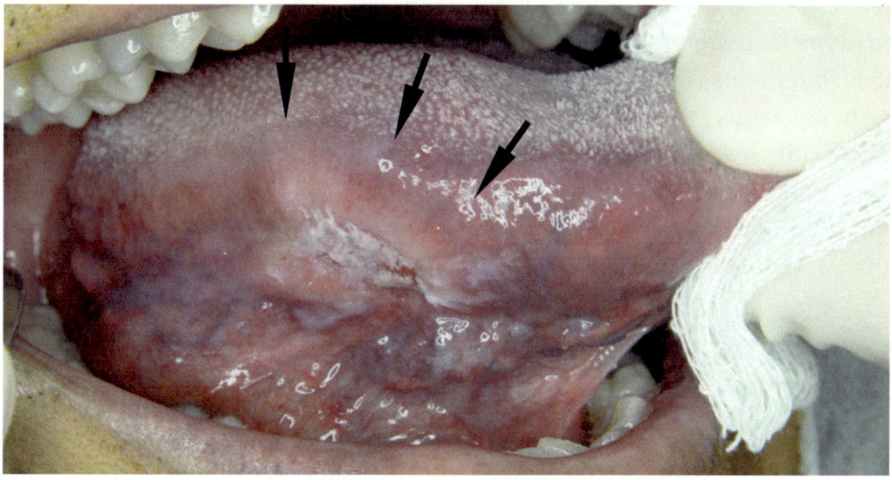

Figure 2. Arrows indicate the lesion showed in Figure 1. Elevated and indurated borders were confirmed by palpation, demonstrating the infiltrative growth of the tumor.

Regarding the symptoms, initial local pain is uncommon [19]. Other signs and symptoms can be dysphagia, weight loss and otalgia (26.5%, 26.6% and 37.5%, respectively) [20], but they seem to be related to the size and anatomic location of the tumor. The duration of the symptoms before diagnosis can vary, but reported data show that most of the patients had early stage disease at the moment of diagnosis, that is, from 52-95% of the patients presented with lesions graded as T1 or T2, usually without neck metastasis [13, 21]. Fang *et al.* [22] reported that 80% of patients younger than 40 years-old with oral SCC presented lesions staged as T1 or T2 and only one tumor with positive node metastasis, appearing to be weakly aggressive at diagnosis. However, the clinical result was poor, as 10 (66.7%) patients exhibited recurrence and five (33%) patients succumbed to the disease [22].

The delay before diagnosis is usually between few weeks and 10 months [23, 24].

3. Microscopic findings

The microscopic features that define an oral SCC do not differ between young and old patients. SCC is an invasive epithelial neoplasm with varying degrees of squamous differentiation. Disorganized stratified squamous epithelium forming strands and islands of bizarre epithelial cells presenting severe dysplasia infiltrating subjacent submucosa is observed. Dyskeratosis, polymorphism, hyperchromatism, atypical mitosis and loss of nucleolus-nucleus and nucleus-cytoplasm ratio are also marked cellular characteristics [25], as shown in Figures 3 and 4.

The tumors are traditionally graded into well, moderately, and poorly differentiated SCC. According to the World Health Organization (WHO), well-differentiated carcinoma resembles closely normal squamous epithelium. Moderately differentiated carcinoma contains distinct nuclear pleomorphism and mitotic activity, including abnormal mitosis, and there is normally less keratinization. In poorly differentiated carcinoma, immature cells predominate, with numerous typical and atypical mitosis, and minimal keratinization. Most of the SCCs are moderately differentiated [25]. The studies in young population also showed a higher incidence of moderately differentiated oral tumors, ranging from 40.9% to 70% of the sample [7, 20, 26-29]. Hilly *et al.* [8] and Garavello *et al.* [27] found worse prognosis and higher indexes of moderately and poor differentiated tumors in their sample. Controversially, Hyam *et al.* [30] found similar prognosis associated with 67% of poorly differentiated tumors. Grading by differentiation is of limited prognostic value, as compared to the pattern of invasion [25].

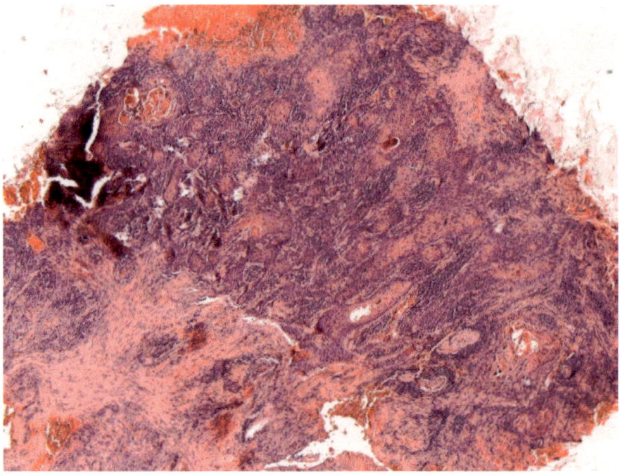

Figure 3. Neoplastic squamous epithelium infiltrating subjacent submucosa (H&E original magnification X50).

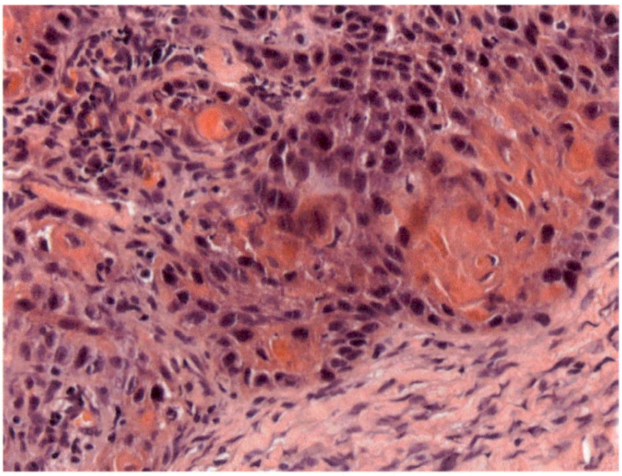

Figure 4. Detail of neoplastic epithelial cells with atypical mitotic figures, dyskeratosis, and loss of nucleolus-nucleus and nucleus-cytoplasm ratio; neoplastic cells presenting polymorphism and hyperchromatism (H&E original magnification X400).

4. Etiology/risk factors

4.1. Tobacco and alcohol

In recent years, an increasing number of young patients, who declare to never having smoked or consumed alcohol excessively, are diagnosed with oral SCC [17, 31]. Tobacco smoke and alcohol abuse are considered well-established risk factors for oral SCC in older population. Otherwise, in young patients, these classical risk factors cannot be considered as the major ones for oral cancer [10, 17, 32, 33], if the period of abuse is not enough to create carcinogenesis [10].

On the other side, some studies report that tobacco use starts during adolescence [10], usually before 16 years old, making probable that before the age of 40 years, patients have an accumulated risk of more than 21 years of consumption, being more susceptible for the oral cancer [34].

Probably, the pathogenesis of oral SCC in young people involves multiple factors, as genetic and others new behavioral factors [32, 33]. It seems that tobacco and alcohol consumption are not the main etiological factors for oral SCC in young patients.

4.2. Genetic factors

Genetic predisposition for cancer development at young age, especially in those patients with no recognized risk factors seems to be preponderant [34]. Chromosome fragility, DNA ploidy abnormalities and increased familial risk of head and neck SCC have already been reported in young patients [26, 34, 35].

Considering the familial risk, a clear significant relative risk of SCC exists in first-degree family members of those who suffered head and neck cancer [35], especially when there is no recognized risk factor associated. Oral cancer has been associated with higher chromosome fragility and instability in youngsters, compared to elderly [36].

Genetic instability is an important molecular mechanism for head and neck cancers [35]. Gain and loss of specific chromosome regions in DNA are responsible for head and neck cancers, for example the 3p or 9p21 region, which are early events strictly related with head and neck cancer development, but that are not commonly seen in young people [35]. It is supposed that a completely different model of tumorigenesis exists, at a molecular level, in young people.

One essential step for tumorigenesis is deregulation of normal cell cycle regulatory system, especially in genes that control G1 to 2 phase progression in cell cycle [37]. The amplification of the gene CCDN1 was noted to be more expressive in young people [31]. CCDN1 is a proto-oncogene that encodes cyclin D1, a key regulator of G1 phase in cell cycle. The overexpression of cyclin D1 was found to be more prominent in young people [31], and it was correlated with disease-free survival in younger and elderly patients. Instead of these findings, larger studies are required to confirm the prognostic value of CCDN1 in young patients.

4.3. Behavioral and other factors

4.3.1. Marijuana consumption

Several cases reported in the literature [38, 39] suggest an association between marijuana smoking and head and neck cancers and respiratory cancers, but this correlation is not conclusive.

The use of marijuana has been speculated as a risk factor for oral cancer in young people [10]. The main reason is that marijuana smoke contains carcinogens similar to those in tobacco, and marijuana smoking involves greater inhalation and longer retention of marijuana smoke [34]. However, the potential of carcinogenicity of tetrahydrocannabiol (THC), the major psychoactive ingredient in marijuana, is not clear yet [40], but it is evident that cannabinoids have an effect in tumorigenic or antitumorigenic role [41]. The patient with oral SCC illustrated in the Figures 1 and 2 confirmed frequent marijuana use when he was a teenager.

4.3.2. Immunodeficiencies

Some chronic immunodeficiency states (Bloom syndrome, Wiskott-Aldrich syndrome), or even immunosuppression regimes following organ transplantation [34] and anemia (Patterson Kelly/ Plummer Vinson syndrome, Fanconi anemia) [35], might play important roles in carcinogenesis in young people. Specifically, Fanconi anemia has an associated higher risk for developing head and neck cancer, estimated to be 40% by the fourth to sixth decade of life. Mutations in telomerase complex are responsible for Fanconi anemia and regarding its malignant transformation, telomeres are repeatedly shortened precipitating a genetic instability, allowing the progression to a malignant neoplasia [35].

Another distinct group that compound young head and neck cancer patients is those with cancer during childhood. The probability of a second synchronous tumor or metachronous primary tumor is estimated in 3–12% in 20 years of survival. Also, chemotherapeutic drugs and radiation can induce malignancies as side effects [7, 42].

4.3.3. Diet

A well-defined concept is that a diet rich in fruits and vegetables, with antioxidant properties, has a protective role against oral cancer [43]. A significant reduction in the risk of oral SCC was found among females consuming three or more portions of fresh fruits and vegetables daily [43, 44]. However, this factor is preponderant for the population in general and there are no studies on specific dietary behavior for young people.

4.3.4. Viral infections

The human papillomavirus (HPV) comprises a huge group of more than 50 subtypes of viruses able to infect the anogenital region and can be divided into two major subgroups: low-risk and high-risk types for cancer [45]. The low-risk HPVs are usually responsible for genital warts that rarely progress into malignancy whereas the high-risk ones have oncogenic capability, leading to the development of cancer. The HPV-16 and HPV-18 are the major high-risk types that are present in anogenital and head and neck cancers [45].

Recent changes in the epidemiological profile of oral carcinoma have encouraged the research for new risk factors related to the development of oral cancer. For example, there has been a decrease in the tobacco-associated oral cancer and an increase of non-smoking white female young patients (18–44 years) who presented with oral SCC [46]. These facts, associated with the established oncogenic power of HPV-16 in cervix carcinoma [47] raised the hypothesis that HPV could be an etiological factor for oral SCC. Moreover, oral mucosa is highly exposed to chemical carcinogens, infections, and trauma, making it more vulnerable to carcinogenesis. Then, it has been postulated that abrasions caused due to this continuous exposure might make this mucosal surface more susceptible to HPV by making it easier for the virus to gain entry into the basal cells of oral mucosa [45].

The mechanism by which the high-risk HPVs promote the carcinogenesis has been already revealed. Once the cell is infected with HPV, the viral oncoproteins E6 and E7 are integrated to the cell genome and their expressions alter the host genome functions [45, 46]. HPV E6 and E7 proteins disrupt p53 and pRb tumor suppressor genes as well as numerous cellular proteins involved in carcinogenesis (BAK, telomerase, INK4A, E2F, cyclins A and E, WAF1, and KIP1) [46]. These accumulated defects in the genomic expression of the infected cells lead to cell immortalization and genomic instability by deactivation of control and regulatory mechanisms of cell apoptosis, cell cycle, and DNA repair [45, 46]. These mechanisms are essential for the development of cervix carcinoma, once HPV prevalence in this type of cancer is 100% [48]. The same is true for oropharyngeal SCC, with a HPV prevalence up to 90% [49, 50]. In oral SCC, the role of HPV still remains unclear. The anatomical structures of oropharynx, especially the base of the tongue and tonsils, seem to be more susceptible to HPV infection when compared to oral sites [34].

The prevalence of HPV in oral cancer may vary from 0 to 100% [51] and this may not be only due to ethno-geographical differences but to the sensitivity of the applied diagnostic technique and to the site of the lesion [51]. The first issue to study the HPV prevalence in these lesions is the techniques employed to detect it. The most accurate ones seem to be the polymerase chain reaction for the HPV DNA and *in situ* hybridization. The immunohistochemistry is also employed but it can lose its accuracy in old specimens [52].

In well-designed studies selected in an elegant review of the literature on the role of HPV in oral SCC, only nine split the groups between young and older people [5, 19, 53-59]. The presence of high-risk HPV had a negative impact for the patient's survival in four studies [5, 19, 55, 58], was neutral in three [53, 54, 59], and had a positive impact in only one investigation [57]. Putting together all data, there is a clear need of more studies with larger samples and more standardized methodology for the virus detection. Despite of the proved role of HPV in the carcinogenesis of the cervix and oropharynx, it is still difficult to draw any conclusion regarding the role of the high-risk HPV types 16 and 18 in the oral cancer development.

5. Treatment

Most cases of oral SCC in young population occur at the mobile tongue. Treatment of tongue tumors at any age depends on the clinical stage at diagnosis. Surgery and radiotherapy are the standards of care for early-stage and also for locally advanced tumors in the oral cavity. The specific treatment is dictated by the TN stage and, if N0 at diagnosis, by the risk of nodal involvement [60]. For T1N0 tumors, surgical resection is recommended and no adjuvant therapy is necessary. The T2 to T4 N0 tumors require local surgery and supraomohyoid neck dissection. Treatment of the neck is expanded according to the worsening of cervical clinical staging. Postoperative radiotherapy is indicated in the following cases: clinical stage III or IV, presence of compromised or small surgical margins, presence of vascular or perineural infiltration, presence of lymph node involvement or extracapsular spread [61]. At present, there is no recommendation for a different approach on oral tumors in young patients [60].

Kaminagakura *et al.* [62] described a better overall survival in a group of young patients (<40-year-old) treated after 1991, when compared to similar patients treated earlier. They attributed this finding to the more aggressive and adequate treatment approaches applied and also to an early diagnosis. So, does the treatment of oral SCC of young people need to be more aggressive? This question can be answered only after understanding the evolution and prognosis of this disease affecting young people. There is a suggestion that people under the age of 40 should be treated differently from the older ones. This is based on the finding of high recurrence and low survival rates between the young. [27]. Also, aggressive therapeutic approach for tongue cancer was recommended by Myers *et al.* [20], with no age distinction. Controversially, Goepfert *et al.* [6] described that young women (<45 years) with oral SCC had similar prognosis when compared to older men and women with this disease, highlighting the unnecessary adoption of adjuvant therapies in this particular group. Is it time to rethink the aggressive treatments and the use of adjuvant unnecessary therapies [21]?

When over treatment occurs in young people, it may be motivated by emotional aspects involving the diagnosis of a lethal condition in such a young person. Also, a radical option may be influenced by the surgeon's experience rather than by scientific evidence [6]. So, it is of utmost importance to know if these tumors have worse prognosis to justify a more aggressive therapy.

6. Prognosis

The outcome for oral SCC occurring in youngsters is a major controversial issue. Various studies have attempted to elucidate the prognostic significance of patient age at diagnosis. Unfortunately, there are no prospective studies comparing elderly and younger patients regarding prognosis. Also, there is no large multicentric research on this topic.

An ordinary question that can greatly affect the results of prognostic studies is the very definition of what would be a young patient with oral SCC. This age limit is empirical and most studies use 40-year-old as the cutoff age [2, 4, 27, 29, 30, 63, 64]. Some outcome analyses use the age of 30, 35, 45 [3, 5-8, 15, 28, 66] or even 60 years as the limit to be considered young [67]. Pediatric patients with oral tumors (under 20 years) have also been studied [9]. So, if there is not much consensus on the age of the patients to be considered young, it is quite difficult to achieve consistent results, regarding the prognosis, when comparing these studies.

Some retrospective reports attempted to analyze prognosis for young population with oral SCC, but they did not compare this data to older counterparts [20, 21, 23, 24, 68-76]. Mallet *et al.* [68] found a high rate of persistent evolution and tumor recurrence within the first year after treatment in a group of patients under 35-year-old, and this affected negatively the overall survival. McGregor *et al.* [24] reported 80% cure rate among patients less than 40 years, but similarly to Mallet *et al.* [68], patients who died from disease usually had a poor response to initial treatment (within the first 2 years). Exceptionally good overall survival for patients < 40 years had been reported [20, 69]. These results suggest a good survival for young patients, albeit with a subgroup of patients developing short term recurrence. The lack of comparison with older counterparts weakened the results, regarding the role of age in prognosis.

The first comparative studies of oral SCC in young and old patients were published in 1998 by Siegelman-Danielli *et al.* [28] and Friedlander *et al.* [2]. They found similar outcome between the groups. Subsequently, another 16 reports compared the evolution of young and older patients with oral SCC, only 4 of them reporting worse prognosis. Analyzing these results, it appears that age at diagnosis has no significance in the outcome for oral SCC.

A matched-pair analysis methodology was performed by some of these comparative reports [2, 3, 5, 6, 15, 27, 62]. This design aims to match similar patients from 2 different groups (old and young), often by sex and disease stage. So, when matched pairs are analyzed, the matched variables are controlled, highlighting the patient's age as an outcome predictor. Only one matched pair analysis [27] showed worse prognosis for young oral cancer patients. This literature is summarized on Table 1.

Although many authors recognized that early age at diagnosis is not an individual factor that worsened outcome, some important information can be extracted from their results. In general, more young patients have recurred locally and regionally [2, 4, 6, 22, 27, 29, 30, 62-64, 65]. This finding may be explained by two theories: lack of adequate treatment and biologically different behavior. Fang *et al.* [22] found 60% of local recurrence in young patients versus 11% among the older ones, and both groups were treated similarly. Another study observed that most of the recurrent young patients had been initially treated with radiotherapy and that this could be the cause for the high recurrence rate [4]. In fact, the reason for inadequate treatment could be explained by the intention to cause less morbidity because of the lower age. Aggressiveness of the surgical procedure is difficult to compare, mainly because it suffers influence of subjective factors during the surgical act and most of the studies had no information about the margin size and status. However, because of the similar treatment approaches used in young and old patients in most of the reports, it is possible that these tumors have a unique biological behavior that needs to be well understood. Siegelmann-Danieli *et al.* [28] reported that tumors developed in the absence of tobacco or alcohol occurred more frequently in young patients and that patients at any age who developed disease without these risk factors may have a worse outcome, reinforcing different pathological behavior.

Authors	Year	Country	Cases/controls	Age limit*	Study Design	Outcome
Siegelmann-Danieli et al.	1998	USA	30/57	45	Non-matched	Similar
Fredlander et al.	1998	USA	36/36	40	Matched-pair analysis	Similar
Pitman et al.	2000	USA	122/150	40	Non-matched	Similar
Vargas et al.	2000	USA	17/17	40	Non-matched	Worse (women)
Hyam et al.	2003	Australia	15/48/60	40	Non-matched	Similar
Veness et al.	2003	Australia	22/142	40	Non-matched	Similar
Popovtzer et al.	2004	Israel	16/32	45	Matched-pair analysis	Similar
Liao et al.	2006	Taiwan	76/220	40	Non-matched	Similar
Siriwardena et al.	2007	Sri Lanka	56/56	40	Non-matched	Similar/ Undefined
Lee et al.	2007	Taiwan	20/20	45	Matched-pair analysis	Better
Garavelo et al.	2007	Italy	46/92	40	Matched-pair analysis	Worse
Ho et al.	2008	Taiwan	28/56	45	Matched-pair analysis	Better
Morris et al.	2010	USA	10/40	20	Non-matched	Similar
Kaminagakura et al.	2010	Brazil	125/250	41	Matched-pair analysis	Similar
Park et al.	2010	Korea	23/62	45	Non-matched	Worse
Soudry et al.	2010	Israel	11/74	30	Non-matched	Similar
Hilly et al.	2013	Israel	16/62	30	Non-matched	Worse when recurrent
Goepfert et al.	2014	USA	18/36	45	Matched-pair analysis	Similar
Fang et al.	2014	China	15/161	40	Non-matched	Similar

*age limit for the young patient's group.

Table 1. Literature review of comparative studies evaluating younger age as a predictor of outcome in oral SCC.

Another interesting fact is that young patients recurred earlier [3, 64] and a high percentage of these recurrent young patients died of their disease [2, 3, 8, 22, 27]. A high index of recurrent disease associated with fatality was observed in the reports of Friedlander *et al.* [2] and Hilly *et al.* [8] (90% and 100%, respectively) and early fatality in 40% was reported by Popovtzer *et al.* [3] (within the two first years).

Moreover, there is some evidence that young patients developed more distant metastasis than the older counterparts [7, 66]. No strong known predicting factors for distant metastasis was found [65] and the observation of 100% incidence of death in distant failure patients indicated that young patients more often present with more advanced disease and may have a distinct pattern of recurrence [7]. Controversially, Fang *et al.* [22] observed 66% of locoregional recurrence without a single distant metastasis in a group of young patients (n=15).

Some recognized microscopic adverse risk features for oral SCC are the extracapsular nodal spread, positive margins, perineural invasion, and vascular embolism [60]. Unfortunately, there is lack of information on microscopic status of the tumors in many reports [3, 5, 9, 63, 64, 66]. Perineural invasion was found to be similar between groups of young and old patients [7, 8]. Siegelmann-Danieli *et al.*[28] found similar extracapsular involvement in both groups, while Hilly *et al.* [8] and Soudry *et al.* [7] found higher, but not significant, index of extracapsular spread in young patients with nodal disease. There is evidence that cellular differentiation, depth of tumor, nerve invasion and extracapsular spread of the involved lymph node were risk factors for distant metastasis in young population with oral cancer. However, these characteristics were not exclusive for young patients [65]. Studies failed to correlate extracapsular involvement, differentiation and perineural invasion to worse outcome in the young [7, 8].

The correlation between the expression of Ki-67, cyclin D1, p16, PCNA, EGFR and angiogenesis with outcome was investigated in young oral cancer population [31, 58, 69, 77, 78]. Overexpression of Ki-67, a cell proliferation marker, was similar in both young and old patients. Angiogenesis also had a similar rate [77]. Moreover, the high expression of cyclin D1 was an indicator of worsened prognosis in both young and old groups [31]. P16 was a marker of favorable prognosis among young population, although not a reliable predictor of HPV presence [58]. A significantly increased number of mitosis, accompanied by strong PCNA expression and higher number of metastasis in the older group were found by Siriwardena *et al.* [78]. The authors believe that oral SCC in the older group is more proliferative, compared with younger patients. Low levels of EGFR expression were associated with lower recurrence rate in young patients, and those with high levels of expression had adverse prognosis [69]. Although there are microscopic factors recognizably influencing prognosis, the available studies failed to demonstrate them in oral cancer affecting young population. These results may be partially explained by the small groups analyzed. The immunoprofile of these tumors are yet to be elucidated, and it appears to be a promising area of research.

A common limitation to all the comparative studies of oral cancer in young people is the small population analyzed, since SCC of the oral cavity is a rare tumor. The largest group of young patients in a single hospital was 125 people at Brazil, but unfortunately the high rates of T3 and T4 disease made this group quite different from the other ones [62]. Pitmann *et al.* [63] studied 122 cases, but their population was not uniform, since 94 of these patients were extracted from previous literature reports. The lower the cutoff age, the lower the sample size. Morris *et al.* [9] and Soudry *et al.* [7] studied only 10 patients (< 20 years) and 11 patients (< 20 years), respectively.

7. Conclusions

Oral SCC in young people accounts for about 0.4–2.6% of the total incidence and has a slight predominance in men. The most common location for this tumor is the tongue and occurrence of symptoms is rare unless the lesion reaches a wide size. The delay before diagnosis varies from few weeks to approximately 10 months.

Concerning the etiological factors for oral SCC in young adults who do not smoke and drink alcohol frequently, genetic abnormalities seem to have a preponderant role in development of the tumor. Additionally, human papilloma virus infection, specifically by HPV-16 and HPV-18, are more frequently detected in this group, but more studies are needed to confirm its influence in prognosis and clinical outcome of oral SCC in the younger.

In the light of current knowledge, it is possible to affirm that age is not an independent outcome predictor for oral SCC. However, a group of young patients that develops a more aggressive disease with a recurrent pattern seems to exist. In this group, early death is common. It is not possible yet to point out the causes for this aggressive behavior. Supported by published studies, treatment should be aggressive for both younger and older patients, and there is no rationale for different approach in young population with oral SCC. Also, further multicentric studies with standardized treatment protocols are necessary in order to elucidate the controversies of this fatal and increasing disease.

Author details

Ligia Buloto Schmitd[1,2], Kellen Cristine Tjioe[1], Agnes Assao[1] and Denise Tostes Oliveira[1*]

*Address all correspondence to: d.tostes@fob.usp.br

1 Department of Stomatology, Pathology Division, Bauru School of Dentistry, University of São Paulo, Bauru, SP, Brazil

2 Department of Stomatology, FAESA Dental School, Vitória, ES, Brazil

References

[1] Patel SC, Carpenter WR, Tyree S, Couch ME, Weissler M, Hackman T, Hayes DN, Shores C, Chera BS. Increasing Incidence of Oral Tongue Squamous Cell Carcinoma in Young White Women, Age 18 to 44 Years. Journal of Clinical Oncology 2011; 29(11) 1488-1494.

[2] Friedlander PL, Schantz SP, Shaha AR, Yu G, Shah JP. Squamous Cell Carcinoma of the Tongue in Young Patients: a Matched-Pair Analysis. Head & Neck 1998; 20(5) 363-368.

[3] Popovtzer A, Shpitzer T, Bahar G, Marshak G, Ulanovski D, Feinmesser R. Squamous Cell Carcinoma of the Oral Tongue in Young Patients. Laryngoscope 2004; 114(5) 915-917.

[4] Siriwardena BS, Tilakaratne A, Amaratunga EA, Tilakaratne WM. Demographic, Aetiological and Survival Differences of Oral Squamous Cell Carcinoma in the Young and the Old in Sri Lanka. Oral Oncology 2006; 42(8) 831-836.

[5] Lee LA, Huang CG, Liao CT, Lee LY, Hsueh C, Chen TC, Lin CY, Fan KH, Wang HM, Huang SF, Chen IH, Kang CJ, Ng SH, Yang SL, Tsao KC, Chang YL, Yen TC. Human Papillomavirus-16 Infection in Advanced Oral Cavity Cancer Patients Is Related to an Increased Risk of Distant Metastases and Poor Survival. PloS One 2012; 7(7) e40767.

[6] Goepfert RP, Kezirian EJ, Wang SJ. Oral Tongue Squamous Cell Carcinoma in Young Women: a Matched Comparison - Do Outcomes Justify Treatment Intensity? ISRN Otolaryngology 2014; 10 ID529395.

[7] Soudry E, Preis M, Hod R, Hamzany Y, Hadar T, Bahar G, Strenov Y, Shpitzer T. Squamous Cell Carcinoma of the Oral Tongue in Patients Younger Than 30 Years: Clinicopathologic Features and Outcome. Clinical Otolaryngology 2010; 35(4) 307-312.

[8] Hilly O, Shkedy Y, Hod R, Soudry E, Mizrachi A, Hamzany Y, Bachar G, Shpitzer T. Carcinoma of the Oral Tongue in Patients Younger Than 30 Years: Comparison with Patients Older Than 60 Years. Oral Oncology 2013; 49(10) 987-990.

[9] Morris LG, Ganly I. Outcomes of Oral Cavity Squamous Cell Carcinoma in Pediatric Patients. Oral Oncology 2010; 46(4) 292-296.

[10] Llewellyn CD, Johnson NW, Warnakulasuriya KA. Risk Factors for Squamous Cell Carcinoma of the Oral Cavity in Young People - a Comprehensive Literature Review. Oral Oncology 2001; 37(5) 401-418.

[11] Halboub E, Al-Mohaya M, Abdulhuq M, Al-Mandili A, Al-Anazi Y. Oral Squamous Cell Carcinoma Among Yemenis: Onset in Young Age and Presentation at Advanced Stage. Journal of Clinical and Experimental Dentistry 2012; 4(4) e221-e225.

[12] Ribeiro AC, Silva AR, Simonato LE, Salzedas LM, Sundefeld ML, Soubhia AM. Clinical and Histopathological Analysis of Oral Squamous Cell Carcinoma in Young People: a Descriptive Study in Brazilians. The British Journal of Oral & Maxillofacial Surgery 2009; 47(2) 95-98.

[13] O'Regan EM, Timon C, Sheils O, Codd M, O'Leary JJ, Toner M. Squamous Cell Carcinoma of the Head and Neck in Young Irish Adults. The British Journal of Oral & Maxillofacial Surgery 2006; 44(3) 203-206.

[14] Shiboski CH, Schmidt BL, Jordan RC. Tongue and Tonsil Carcinoma: Increasing Trends in the U.S. Population Ages 20-44 Years. Cancer 2005; 103(9) 1843-1849.

[15] Ho HC, Lee MS, Hsiao SH, Hwang JH, Hung SK, Chou P, Lee CC. Squamous Cell Carcinoma of the Oral Cavity in Young Patients: a Matched-Pair Analysis. European Archives of Oto-Rhino-Laryngology 2008; 265(1 Suppl) S57-S61.

[16] Udeabor SE, Rana M, Wegener G, Gellrich NC, Eckardt AM. Squamous Cell Carcinoma of the Oral Cavity and the Oropharynx in Patients Less Than 40 Years of Age: a 20-Year Analysis. Head & Neck Oncology 2012; 4 28.

[17] Kuriakose M, Sankaranarayanan M, Nair MK, Cherian T, Sugar AW, Scully C, Prime SS. Comparison of Oral Squamous Cell Carcinoma in Younger and Older Patients in India. European Journal of Cancer, Part B. Oral Oncology 1992; 28B(2) 113-120.

[18] Falaki F, Dalirsani Z, Pakfetrat A, Falaki A, Saghravanian N, Nosratzehi T, Pazouki M. Clinical and Histopathological Analysis of Oral Squamous Cell Carcinoma of Young Patients in Mashhad, Iran: a Retrospective Study and Review of Literature. Medicina Oral, Patologia Oral y Cirugia Bucal 2011; 16(4) e473-e477.

[19] Sharma A, Mendez E, Yueh B, Lohavanichbutr P, Houck J, Doody DR, Futran ND, Upton MP, Schwartz SM, Chen C. Human Papillomavirus-Positive Oral Cavity and Oropharyngeal Cancer Patients Do Not Have Better Quality-of-Life Trajectories. Otolaryngology - Head and Neck Surgery 2012; 146(5) 739-745.

[20] Myers JN, Elkins T, Roberts D, Byers RM. Squamous Cell Carcinoma of the Tongue in Young Adults: Increasing Incidence and Factors that Predict Treatment Outcomes. Otolaryngology - Head and Neck Surgery 2000; 122(1) 44-51.

[21] Manuel S, Raghavan SK, Pandey M, Sebastian P. Survival in Patients Under 45 Years with Squamous Cell Carcinoma of the Oral Tongue. International Journal of Oral and Maxillofacial Surgery 2003; 32(2) 167-173.

[22] Fang QG, Shi S, Liu FY, Sun CF. Tongue Squamous Cell Carcinoma as a Possible Distinct Entity in Patients Under 40 Years Old. Oncology Letters 2014; 7(6) 2099-2102.

[23] Venables CW, Craft IL. Carcinoma of the Tongue in Early Adult Life. British Journal of Cancer 1967; 21(4) 645-650.

[24] McGregor GI, Davis N, Robins RE. Squamous Cell Carcinoma of the Tongue and Lower Oral Cavity in Patients Under 40 Years of Age. American Journal of Surgery 1983; 146(1) 88-92.

[25] Barnes L, Everson JW, Reichart P, Sidransky D. World Health Organization Classification of Tumors. Pathology and Genetics of Head and Neck Tumors. IARC Press: Lyon 2005.

[26] Santos-Silva AR, Ribeiro AC, Soubhia AM, Miyahara GI, Carlos R, Speight PM, Hunter KD, Torres-Rendon A, Vargas PA, Lopes MA. High Incidences of DNA Ploidy Abnormalities in Tongue Squamous Cell Carcinoma of Young Patients: an International Collaborative Study. Histopathology 2011; 58(7) 1127-1135.

[27] Garavello W, Spreafico R, Gaini RM. Oral Tongue Cancer in Young Patients: a Matched Analysis. Oral Oncology 2007; 43(9) 894-897.

[28] Siegelmann-Danieli N, Hanlon A, Ridge JA, Padmore R, Fein DA, Langer CJ. Oral Tongue Cancer in Patients Less Than 45 Years Old: Institutional Experience and Comparison with Older Patients. Journal of Clinical Oncology 1998; 16(2) 745-753.

[29] Veness MJ, Morgan GJ, Sathiyaseelan Y, Gebski V. Anterior Tongue Cancer: Age Is Not a Predictor of Outcome and Should Not Alter Treatment. ANZ Journal of Surgery 2003; 73(11) 899-904.

[30] Hyam DM, Conway RC, Sathiyaseelan Y, Gebski V, Morgan GJ, Walker DM, Veness MJ. Tongue Cancer: do Patients Younger Than 40 Do Worse? Australian Dental Journal 2003; 48(1) 50-54.

[31] Kaminagakura E, Werneck da Cunha I, Soares FA, Nishimoto IN, Kowalski LP. CCND1 Amplification and Protein Overexpression in Oral Squamous Cell Carcinoma of Young Patients. Head & Neck 2011; 33(10) 1413-1419.

[32] Bodner E, Palgi Y, Kaveh D. Does the Relationship Between Affect Complexity and Self-esteem Differ in Young-Old and Old-Old Participants? The Journals of Gerontology. Series B, Psychological Sciences and Social Sciences 2013; 68(5) 665-673.

[33] Turi K, Barabas P, Csurgay K, Lehner GY, Lorincz A, Nemeth ZS. An Analysis of the Epidemiological and Etiological Factors of Oral Tumors of Young Adults in a Central-Eastern European Population. Pathology & Oncology Research 2013; 19(3) 353-363.

[34] Majchrzak E, Szybiak B, Wegner A, Pienkowski P, Pazdrowski J, Luczewski L, Sowka M, Golusinski P, Malicki J, Golusinski W. Oral Cavity and Oropharyngeal Squamous Cell Carcinoma in Young Adults: a Review of the Literature. Radiology and Oncology 2014; 48(1) 1-10.

[35] Toner M, O'Regan EM. Head and Neck Squamous Cell Carcinoma in the Young: a Spectrum or a Distinct Group? Part 1. Head and Neck Pathology 2009; 3(3) 246-248.

[36] Kostrzewska-Poczekaj M, Gawecki W, Illmer J, Rydzanicz M, Gajecka M, Szyfter W, Szyfter K. Polymorphisms of DNA Repair Genes and Risk of Squamous Cell Carcinoma of the Head and Neck in Young Adults. European Archives of Oto-Rhino-Laryngology 2013; 270(1) 271-276.

[37] Scully C, Field JK, Tanzawa H. Genetic Aberrations in Oral or Head and Neck Squamous Cell Carcinoma (SCCHN): 1. Carcinogen Metabolism, DNA Repair and Cell Cycle Control. Oral Oncology 2000; 36(3) 256-263.

[38] Zhang ZF, Morgenstern H, Spitz MR, Tashkin DP, Yu GP, Marshall JR, Hsu TC, Schantz SP. Marijuana Use and Increased Risk of Squamous Cell Carcinoma of the Head and Neck. Cancer Epidemiology, Biomarkers & Prevention 1999; 8(12) 1071-1078.

[39] Hashibe M, Ford DE, Zhang ZF. Marijuana Smoking and Head and Neck Cancer. Journal of Clinical Pharmacology 2002; 42(11 Suppl) 103S-107S.

[40] Guzman M. Cannabinoids: Potential Anticancer Agents. Nature Reviews. Cancer 2003; 3(11) 745-755.

[41] Liang C, McClean MD, Marsit C, Christensen B, Peters E, Nelson HH, Kelsey KT. A Population-Based Case-Control Study of Marijuana Use and Head and Neck Squamous Cell Carcinoma. Cancer Prevention Research 2009; 2(8) 759-768.

[42] Curado MP, Hashibe M. Recent Changes in the Epidemiology of Head and Neck Cancer. Current Opinion in Oncology 2009; 21(3) 194-200.

[43] Llewellyn CD, Linklater K, Bell J, Johnson NW, Warnakulasuriya S. An Analysis of Risk Factors for Oral Cancer in Young People: a Case-Control Study. Oral Oncology 2004 Mar; 40(3) 304-313.

[44] Rodriguez T, Altieri A, Chatenoud L, Gallus S, Bosetti C, Negri E, Franceschi S, Levi F, Talamini R, La Vecchia C. Risk Factors for Oral and Pharyngeal Cancer in Young Adults. Oral Oncology 2004; 40(2) 207-213.

[45] Chocolatewala NM, Chaturvedi P. Role of Human Papilloma Virus in the Oral Carcinogenesis: an Indian Perspective. Journal of Cancer Research and Therapeutics 2009; 5(2) 71-77.

[46] Kansy K, Thiele O, Freier K. The Role of Human Papillomavirus in Oral Squamous Cell Carcinoma: Myth and Reality. Oral and Maxillofacial Surgery 2014; 18(2) 165-172.

[47] Durst M, Gissmann L, Ikenberg H, zur Hausen H. A Papillomavirus DNA from a Cervical Carcinoma and Its Prevalence in Cancer Biopsy Samples from Different Geographic Regions. Proceedings of the National Academy of Sciences of the United States of America 1983; 80(12) 3812-3815.

[48] Stanley M. Pathology and Epidemiology of HPV Infection in Females. Gynecologic Oncology 2010; 117(2 Suppl) S5-S10.

[49] Gillison ML, Koch WM, Capone RB, Spafford M, Westra WH, Wu L, Zahurak ML, Daniel RW, Viglione M, Symer DE, Shah KV, Sidransky D. Evidence for a Causal As-

sociation Between Human Papillomavirus and a Subset of Head and Neck Cancers. Journal of the National Cancer Institute 2000; 92(9) 709-720.

[50] Marur S, D'Souza G, Westra WH, Forastiere AA. HPV-Associated Head and Neck Cancer: a Virus-Related Cancer Epidemic. The Lancet Oncology 2010; 11(8) 781-789.

[51] Termine N, Panzarella V, Falaschini S, Russo A, Matranga D, Lo Muzio L, Campisi G. HPV in Oral Squamous Cell Carcinoma vs Head and Neck Squamous Cell Carcinoma Biopsies: a Meta-Analysis (1988-2007). Annals of Oncology 2008; 19(10) 1681-1690.

[52] Kaminagakura E, Villa LL, Andreoli MA, Sobrinho JS, Vartanian JG, Soares FA, Nishimoto IN, Rocha R, Kowalski LP. High-Risk Human Papillomavirus in Oral Squamous Cell Carcinoma of Young Patients. International Journal of Cancer 2012; 130(8) 1726-1732.

[53] Campisi G, Giovannelli L, Calvino F, Matranga D, Colella G, Di Liberto C, Capra G, Leao JC, Lo Muzio L, Capogreco M, D'Angelo M. HPV Infection in Relation to OSCC Histological Grading and TNM Stage. Evaluation by Traditional Statistics and Fuzzy Logic Model. Oral Oncology 2006; 42(6) 638-645.

[54] D'Souza G, Zhang HH, D'Souza WD, Meyer RR, Gillison ML. Moderate Predictive Value of Demographic and Behavioral Characteristics for a Diagnosis of HPV16-Positive and HPV16-Negative Head and Neck Cancer. Oral Oncology 2010; 46(2) 100-104.

[55] Duray A, Descamps G, Decaestecker C, Remmelink M, Sirtaine N, Lechien J, Ernoux-Neufcoeur P, Bletard N, Somja J, Depuydt CE, Delvenne P, Saussez S. Human Papillomavirus DNA Strongly Correlates with a Poorer Prognosis in Oral Cavity Carcinoma. The Laryngoscope 2012; 122(7) 1558-1565.

[56] El-Mofty SK, Lu DW. Prevalence of Human Papillomavirus Type 16 DNA in Squamous Cell Carcinoma of the Palatine Tonsil, and Not the Oral Cavity, in Young Patients: a Distinct Clinicopathologic and Molecular Disease Entity. The American Journal of Surgical Pathology 2003; 27(11) 1463-1470.

[57] Gillison ML, D'Souza G, Westra W, Sugar E, Xiao W, Begum S, Viscidi R. Distinct Risk Factor Profiles for Human Papillomavirus Type 16-Positive and Human Papillomavirus Type 16-Negative Head and Neck Cancers. Journal of the National Cancer Institute 2008; 100(6) 407-420.

[58] Harris SL, Thorne LB, Seaman WT, Hayes DN, Couch ME, Kimple RJ. Association of p16(INK4a) Overexpression with Improved Outcomes in Young Patients with Squamous Cell Cancers of the Oral Tongue. Head & Neck 2011; 33(11) 1622-1627.

[59] Marques-Silva L, Farias LC, Fraga CA, de Oliveira MV, Cardos CM, Fonseca-Silva T, Gomes CC, De-Paula AM, Gomez RS, Guimaraes AL. HPV-16/18 Detection Does Not Affect the Prognosis of Head and Neck Squamous Cell Carcinoma in Younger and Older Patients. Oncology Letters 2012; 3(4) 945-949.

[60] NCCN Clinical Practice Guidelines in Oncology. Head and Neck Cancers Version 2.2014. http://www.nccn.org/professionals/physician_gls/pdf/head-and-neck.pdf

[61] Kowalsky LP, Carvalho AL, Pellizon ACA. Carcinoma de Boca. In: Kowalsky LP *et al.* (Eds.) Manual de Condutas Diagnósticas e Terapêuticas em Oncologia. Ambito Editores: São Paulo 2002. pp. 411-416.

[62] Kaminagakura E, Vartanian JG, Silva SD, Santos CR, Kowalski LP. Case Control Study on Prognostic Factors in Oral Squamous Cell Carcinoma in Young Patients. Head & Neck 2010; 32(11) 1460-1466.

[63] Pitman KT, Johnson JT, Wagner RL, Myers EN. Cancer of the Tongue in Patients Less Than Forty. Head & Neck 2000; 22(3) 297-302.

[64] Vargas H, Pitman KT, Johnson JT, Galati LT. More Aggressive Behavior of Squamous Cell Carcinoma of the Anterior Tongue in Young Women. Laryngoscope 2000; 110(10 Pt 1) 1623-1626.

[65] Park JO, Sun DI, Cho KJ, Joo YH, Yoo HJ, Kim MS. Clinical Outcome of Squamous Cell Carcinoma of the Tongue in Young Patients: a Stage-Matched Comparative Analysis. Clinical and Experimental Otorhinolaryngology 2010; 3(3) c161-c165.

[66] Liao CT, Wang HM, Hsieh LL, Chang JT, Ng SH, Hsueh C, Lee LY, Lin CH, Chen IH, Kang CJ, Huang SF, Yen TC. Higher Distant Failure in Young Age Tongue Cancer Patients. Oral Oncology 2006; 42(7) 718-725.

[67] Vered M, Dayan D, Dobriyan A, Yahalom R, Shalmon B, Barshack I, Bedrin L, Talmi YP, Taicher S. Oral Tongue Squamous Cell Carcinoma: Recurrent Disease Is Associated with Histopathologic Risk Score and Young Age. Journal of Cancer Research and Clinical Oncology 2010; 136(7) 1039-1048.

[68] Mallet Y, Avalos N, Le Ridant AM, Gangloff P, Moriniere S, Rame JP, Poissonnet G, Makeieff M, Cosmidis A, Babin E, Barry B, Fournier C. Head and Neck Cancer in Young People: a Series of 52 SCCs of the Oral Tongue in Patients Aged 35 Years or Less. Acta Oto-Laryngologica 2009; 129(12) 1503-1508.

[69] Thomas L, Moore EJ, McGree ME, Olsen KD, Kasperbauer JL, Erickson LA, Schembri-Wismayer DJ. Prognostic Features, Human Papillomavirus Status, and Epidermal Growth Factor Receptor Expression in Oral Squamous Cell Carcinoma in Young Adults. American Journal of Otolaryngology 2012; 33(6) 650-656.

[70] Sarkaria JN, Harari PM. Oral Tongue Cancer in Young Adults Less Than 40 Years of Age: Rationale for Aggressive Therapy. Head & Neck 1994; 16(2) 107-111.

[71] Brägelmann J, Dagogo-Jack I, El Dinali M, Stricker T, Brown CD, Zuo Z, Khattri A, Keck M, McNerney ME, Longnecker R, Bieging K, Kocherginsky M, Alexander K, Salgia R, Lingen MW, Vokes EE, White KP, Cohen EE, Seiwert TY. Oral Cavity Tumors in Younger Patients Show a Poor Prognosis and Do Not Contain Viral RNA. Oral Oncology 2013; 49(6) 525-533.

[72] Newman AN, Rice DH, Ossoff RH, Sisson GA. Carcinoma of the Tongue in Persons Younger Than 30 Years of Age. Archives of Otolaryngology 1983; 109(5) 302-304.

[73] Amsterdam JT, Strawitz JG. Squamous Cell Carcinoma of the Oral Cavity in Young Adults. Journal of Surgical Oncology 1982; 19(2) 65-68.

[74] Iype EM, Pandey M, Mathew A, Thomas G, Nair MK. Squamous Cell Cancer of the Buccal Mucosa in Young Adults. The British Journal of Oral and Maxillofacial Surgery 2004; 42(3) 185-189.

[75] Byers RM. Squamous Cell Carcinoma of the Oral Tongue in Patients Less Than Thirty Years of Age. The American Journal of Surgery 1975; 130(4) 475-478.

[76] Davidson BJ, Root WA, Trock BJ. Age and Survival from Squamous Cell Carcinoma of the Oral Tongue. Head & Neck 2001; 23(4) 273-279.

[77] Benevenuto TG, Nonaka CF, Pinto LP, de Souza LB. Immunohistochemical Comparative Analysis of Cell Proliferation and Angiogenic Index in Squamous Cell Carcinomas of the Tongue Between Young and Older Patients. Applied Immunohistochemistry & Molecular Morphology 2012; 20(3) 291-297.

[78] Siriwardena BS, Tilakaratne A, Amaratunga EA, Udagama MN, Ogawa I, Kudo Y, Takata T, Tilakaratne WM. Analysis of Histopathological and Immunohistochemical Differences of Oral Squamous Cell Carcinoma in Young and Old Patients in Sri Lanka. Journal of Oral Pathology & Medicine 2007; 36(6) 357-362.

Chapter 6

Local Metastasis in Head and Neck Cancer - an Overview

Suwarna Dangore–Khasbage

Additional information is available at the end of the chapter

http://dx.doi.org/10.5772/60072

1. Introduction

Head and neck cancer refers to epithelial malignancies of various parts of the orofacial region, which include paranasal sinuses, nasal cavity, pharynx and larynx, etc. These represent about 6% of all cancer cases and account for a number of new cancer cases and cancer-related deaths worldwide every year [1, 2]. Amongst those, oral cancer is the most common type of cancer. Squamous cell carcinoma is the most frequent single entity, constituting 95% of all oral malignancies [3].

Oral squamous cell carcinoma is an invasive lesion with the presence of perineural growth. It has a significant recurrence rate and frequently metastasizes to cervical lymph nodes. Since squamous cell carcinoma constitutes the preponderance of primary malignancies of the head and neck, it is by far the most common tumour that spreads to the cervical nodes [4]. Reports from the American Cancer Society indicate that, at the time of initial diagnosis, over 40% of patients with squamous cell carcinomas of the oral cavity and pharynx present with regional dissemination of the disease [5].

In oral cancer, tumour dissemination occurs via regional lymphatic to cervical lymph node in a predictable and sequential fashion. Oral cancer occurring in the posterior aspect of the oral cavity, oropharynx and inferior of the mouth tends to be associated with a higher incidence of spread to the lymph nodes at the time of diagnosis. Ipsilateral lymph nodes metastases are frequent. However, its spreading to contralateral nodes is more common with midline and posterior lesions [6].

The incidence of spread is influenced by the size of the tumour. Lesions classed as T1 may show a regional spread in 10 to 20% of cases, T2 lesions in 25 to 30% of cases and T3 to T4 tumours in 50 to 75% [6].

The determination of the presence or absence of metastases in the neck nodes is mandatory for cancer-bearing patients. This is because the therapeutic rational and prognosis depend on the staging of the cancer. It is stated that the presence of metastatic node reduces the 5-year survival rate by 50%. Moreover, the presence of another metastatic node on the contralateral side further reduces the survival rate by 25% [7]. Patients with metastasis need more aggressive treatments. Therefore, it is important to assess as reliably as possible whether or not a patient has regional lymph node metastases.

The common cause of metastatic cervical lymphadenopathy is the spread from primary tumours in the head and neck region. However, in unusual cases, they represent secondary tumours from primary sites below the clavicles [3]. The diagnosis of such cervical neck tumours can be decided after a complete clinical and radiological examination, focusing on the organs or areas where there is a high chance of an existing primary tumour.

2. Mechanism of metastases in head and neck cancer

The most deadly aspect of any cancer is its ability to spread or metastasize. Metastasis is a complex process involving the detachment of cells from the tumour tissue, the regulation of cell motility and invasion, and the proliferation and evasion through the lymphatic system or blood vessels.

There are different views regarding the involvement of regional lymph nodes in metastasis. The nearby lymph nodes in tumour-bearing hosts are considered as anatomic barriers to the spread of tumour cells. On the contrary, another concept is that the lymphatic and lymphaticovenous shunts bypass the regional lymph nodes and allow both the lymphatic and haematogenous dissemination of malignant cells. [8].

Cancer cells have the ability to overcome the safeguards that are present in the body for the prevention of metastasis. It is necessary to understand what ways cancer cells have mutated in order to circumvent the body's defences and travel freely to other locations.

2.1. Lymphatic drainage in head and neck cancer

Several important groups of lymph nodes act as first echelon nodes of the oral cavity. The first lymph node encountered in the channel, which drains a particular submucosal or subepidermal lymph capillary plexus, is called the first echelon node. This is because it is here that pathogenic organisms or free tumour cells within the lymph fluid meet their first resistance to travel. A sentinel lymph node is defined as the first lymph node in a regional lymphatic basin that receives lymph flow from the primary tumour. Sentinel node imaging provides a "road map" of the lymphatic drainage from a tumour. However, it does not provide information regarding the presence or absence of cancer cells in those nodes.

Sometimes, lymphatic metastases do not first develop in the lymph nodes nearest to the tumour. This is known as skip metastases. The reason for this phenomenon could be venous lymphatic anastomoses or obliteration of lymphatics by inflammation or radiation. Due to the obstruction of the lymphatics by tumour cells, the lymph flow is disturbed and the tumour cells spread against the flow of the lymph. This causes retrograde metastases at unusual sites, for example, metastases of carcinoma prostrate to the supraclavicular nodes. It is believed that lymph nodes in the vicinity of the tumour perform multiple roles – first, acting as an initial barrier filter and destructing tumour cells, while later providing fertile soil for the growth of tumour cells [9].

Cervical lymph nodes include the submental, prevascular facial and submandibular group of lymph nodes. Deep jugular lymph nodes include the jugulodigastric, juguloomohyoid and supraclavicular group of lymph nodes. Lymph nodes in the posterior triangle of the neck include the accessory chain of lymph nodes. The mucosa of the upper aerodigestive tract drains to the cervical lymph nodes in the lateral aspect of the neck. Tumours of the pharynx may drain to the parapharyngeal and retropharyngeal lymph nodes.

The Delphian lymph node is present in the central compartment of the neck and drains the larynx and perithyroid lymph nodes adjacent to the thyroid gland. Lymph nodes in the tracheoesophageal groove provide primary drainage to the thyroid gland, as well as the hypopharynx, subglottic larynx and cervical oesophagus. Lymph nodes in the anterior superior mediastinum provide drainage to the thyroid gland and the oesophagus. Furthermore, they serve as a secondary lymphatic basin for anatomic structures in the central compartment of the neck. Each anatomic subgroup of lymph nodes described above specifically serve as primary echelon lymph nodes, draining a specific site in the head and neck region. Thus, the location of a palpable metastatic lymph node may often indicate the source of a primary tumour [8].

2.2. Assumptions about the mechanism of metastases

Lymph node metastasis occurs by haematogenous or by lymphatic routes. The cancer mass has the same vascularity as that of healthy tissue. Thus, the cancer cells have access to the blood stream. The malignant cells are detached from the tumour mass and enter the body's circulation. Once in the bloodstream, the cancer cells circulate to other parts of the body. Similarly, the lymphatic system has channels throughout the body, like the circulatory system, through which a malignant cell can travel and metastasize.

If the cells travel through the lymph system, they may end up in nearby lymph nodes or spread to other organs. In circulation, the cancer cells may reach to any part of the body where they begin to grow and form a secondary tumour mass. This spread of cancer to a new part of the body is called metastasis. The spread of malignancy to nearby lymph nodes is called local or regional metastasis and the spread of the tumour to a distant organ is called a distant metastasis.

Cancer cells have to go through several steps in order to spread to new parts of the body:

a. The loose cancer cells have to be able to break away from the parent tumour.

b. They have to gain entry into the bloodstream or lymph system - this can carry them to another part of the body.

c. They have to attach to the wall of a blood vessel or lymph vessel.

d. They need to survive in a blood vessel or lymph vessel and move through it into a new organ.

e. Malignant cells have to emerge from a blood or lymph vessel.

f. They need to be able to multiply and grow to form secondary neoplasm at the new site.

g. They need to be able to avoid attacks from the body's immune system.

There are various factors that may influence the mechanism of regional metastases and prevent tumour cells from developing lymph node metastases. These are:

1. The suppression of cellular immune response, in particular T cell function [7].

2. The microvascular invasion, grade of differentiation and tumour thickness in metastases of squamous cell carcinoma of the oral cavity [10].

3. The lymphatic vessel in and around the tumour tissue and lymph node metastasis in patients with oral squamous cell carcinoma. The dimension of lymphatic vessels is significantly greater in the tumour tissue than in the tumour-free tissue. This means that the function of lymphatic vessels appear to have increased in the tumour tissue, compared to the tumour-free tissue. This results in regional metastasis [11].

Reviews of literature recommend that there are multiple and diverse reasons for cervical lymph node metastases in head and neck cancer. However, by any means, the careful evaluation of these metastatic regional nodes is essential for appropriate treatment and to achieve the best outcome of the treatment. Certainly, a careful clinical examination must be carried out at the beginning of the journey regarding the evaluation of the status of cervical lymph nodes in head and neck cancer.

3. Clinical examination of lymph nodes in head and neck cancer

Customarily, all of the palpable cervical lymph nodes are considered as positive for regional metastasis in oral cancer. Thus, to treat all necks by considering the significant risk of having occult lymph node metastases is a traditional approach for the treatment of oral cancer. However, this approach often involves the unnecessary treatment of necks that ultimately prove to be pathologically free of cancer. Therefore, appropriate investigations should be carried out. These will help to determine the treatment plan, prognosis and morbidity by diminishing the possibility of unnecessary neck dissection.

The location, number, size, shape, tenderness, consistency and fixity to underlying structures are the criteria routinely used during a clinical examination of the cervical lymph nodes.

Usually, a 1 cm size cut-off in the largest axial diameter is used for metastatic disease. However, size is not a reliable marker of malignancy as small nodes can harbour small metastases that do not expand the node and conversely, benign nodes can be enlarged due to hyperplasia or inflammation. Thus, the nodes of less than 1 cm should also be carefully evaluated, particularly if they are in expected drainage sites of the primary tumour. In clinical practice, the size of the lymph node is only considered useful when there is an increase in nodal size on serial examinations in a patient with a known primary tumour, which is highly suggestive of metastasis.

Metastatic disease can change the shape of the node by infiltrating nodal tissue and expanding the nodal capsule. Rounded nodes are more suspicious than oval nodes. As the disease progresses, ill-defined irregular margins in a lymph node are a sign of malignancy and may represent an extracapsular spread of tumour.

Metastatic lymph nodes are usually painless and thus, remain undetected by the patient until they reach considerable dimensions. Characteristically, these nodes are stony-hard and freely movable until the tumour cells penetrate the node capsule and invade the surrounding tissue. Then, they become fixed and the expanding tumour may amalgamate surrounding nodes into one larger, stony-hard and fixed mass. Sometimes, the small tumours in the nasal cavities, nasopharynx and larynx may go undetected. The only evidence of their presence is the metastatic tumour.

Oral cavity tumours usually cause metastasis in the submandibular and upper cervical regions. Rarely, lymph nodes in the posterior triangle may also be involved. The malignancy of the tongue base and tonsillar fossa is often the reason for metastatic lymphadenopathy in the posterior triangle of neck.

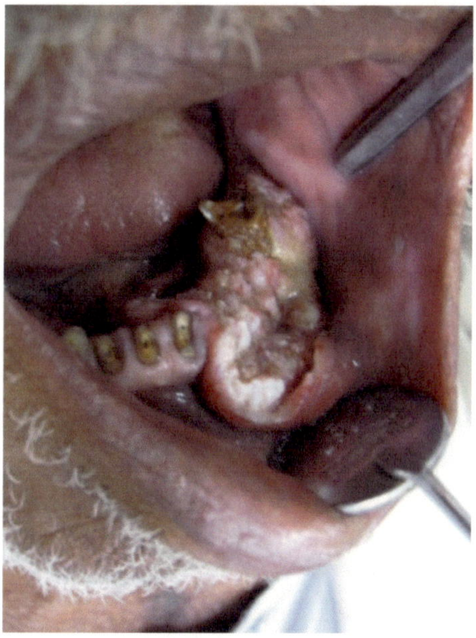

Figure 1. Ulceroproliferative growth with rolled edges, involving buccal and lingual vestibule and alveolar ridge in a 62-year-old male. There was a history of tobacco-lime quid keeping in the same region since 30 years of age.

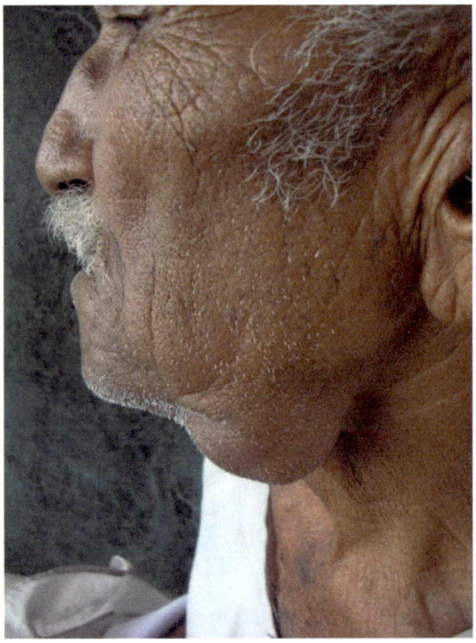

Figure 2. Showing an enlarged (4 × 4 cm), hard and fixed submandibular lymph node in a patient with a malignancy of bucco- lingual vestibule and alveolar ridge (extra oral photograph of the same 62-year-old male, shown in Figure 1)

4. Clinical staging of cervical lymph nodes in head and neck cancer

In the 1940s, the tumour-node-metastasis (TNM) staging system was reported by Pierre Denoix. The TNM staging system is an anatomic staging system that describes the anatomic extent of the primary tumour, the involvement of regional lymph nodes and distant metastasis.

As head and neck cancers consist of tumours arising from a variety of anatomic sites, such as the oral cavity, nasal cavity, paranasal sinuses, nasopharynx, oropharynx, hypopharynx, larynx, oesophagus, thyroid gland, salivary glands, etc., and miscellaneous tumours, such as neurogenic tumours, it is impossible to generate a uniform staging system that would be relevant for all tumours arising in the head and neck region. In current practice, information obtained from the clinical examination and radiologic imaging is used to assign a clinical stage (cTNM). This is then used to stratify patients for a selection of therapy and to report outcomes of the treatment.

For many decades, the AJCC-UICC TNM staging system has been used worldwide for staging head and neck cancer [12, 13]. This system has been periodically revised for improvement. According to this, the cervical lymph nodes are divided into seven levels or groups, which are based on the extent and level of cervical nodal involvement by metastatic tumour. Although this classification of cervical lymph nodes is commonly used, especially by surgeons and oncologists, some important lymph nodes, such as parotid and retropharyngeal nodes, are not included in this classification.

Stage	Criteria
Nx	Regional lymph nodes cannot be assessed.
No	No regional lymph node metastasis.
N1	Metastasis in a single ipsilateral lymph node, < 3 cm in greatest dimension.
N2a	Metastasis in a single ipsilateral lymph node, > 3 cm but < 6 cm in greatest dimension.
N2b	Metastasis in multiple ipsilateral lymph nodes, none > 6 cm in greatest dimension.
N2c	Metastasis in bilateral or contralateral lymph nodes, none > 6 cm in greatest dimension.
N3	Metastasis in a lymph node > 6 cm in greatest dimension.

Table 1. N staging for all Head and neck sites except the nasopharynx and thyroid - AJCC/UICC 2002 [12, 13].

Stage	Criteria
Nx	Regional lymph nodes cannot be assessed.
No	No regional lymph node metastasis.
N1	Unilateral metastasis in lymph node(s), 6 cm or less in greatest dimension, above the supraclavicular fossa.*
N2	Bilateral metastasis in lymph node(s), 6 cm or less in greatest dimension, above the supraclavicular fossa. *
N3	Metastasis in a lymph node(s) > 6 cm and/or to supraclavicular fossa.
N3a	Greater than 6 cm in dimension.
N3b	Extension to the supraclavicular fossa. *

*Midline nodes are considered ipsilateral nodes.

Table 2. N staging for tumours of the nasopharynx - AJCC/UICC 2002 [12, 13].

Stage	Criteria
Nx	Regional lymph nodes cannot be assessed.*
No	No regional lymph node metastasis.
N1	Regional lymph node metastasis.
N1a	Metastasis to Level VI (pretracheal, paratracheal and prelaryngeal/Delphian lymph nodes).
N1b	Metastasis to unilateral, bilateral, or contralateral cervical or superior mediastinal lymph nodes.

*Regional nodes are the central compartment, lateral cervical, and upper mediastinal lymph nodes.

Table 3. N staging for tumours of the thyroid - AJCC/UICC 2002 [12, 13].

The **TNM** staging system is widely used to assess prognosis, determine treatment and compare results from different protocols. However, it has a few pitfalls. The palpable lymph node in the neck does not always mean that it is metastatic and a non-palpable does not always mean that it is non-metastatic. They may contain micrometastases and may be discovered on a histological examination, which were thought to be normal on palpation and imaging.

One or more non-painful nodes in asymptomatic patients or patients with an already diagnosed malignancy in the T1-T2 stage in satellite or non-satellite locations are considered as risky nodes. Furthermore, in patients with an already diagnosed malignancy in the T3-T4 stage, three or more > 2 cm nodes in a satellite location are called end–stage nodes [14].

TNM staging systems are based on clinical findings. However, imaging should be a necessary part of this staging or it should always be used to support the staging. If the imaging complements the clinical examination, the following staging conversions can occur: N0 will become N1 neck, N1 will become N2 neck, N1 will become N3c neck or N0 will become N3c neck [15].

5. Diagnosis and investigations for metastatic lymph nodes in head and neck cancer

Imaging plays an important role in the evaluation of disease in the cervical lymph nodes and should be a part of any thorough workup of patients with head and neck cancer. The continuous advances in techniques have led to the increased sensitivity of the imaging modalities in the detection of lymph nodes. Various imaging techniques are used for the detection of enlarged nodes, including ultrasound, Colour Doppler ultrasound, computed tomography, magnetic resonance imaging positron emission tomography (PET), lymphoscintigraphy and USG-guided fine-needle cytology, etc. Each imaging modality has advantages and disadvantages [16].

5.1. Ultrasound and colour doppler ultrasound examination of neck in head and neck cancer

Ultrasound (US) is a non-invasive, easily accessible and comparatively cheaper imaging modality, which is used for the evaluation of cervical lymphadenopathy. The sonologist is often the first person to identify the presence of an abnormal node. Several studies have shown that sonography has a markedly higher sensitivity than palpation for the detection of enlarged lymph nodes in patients with suspected regional lymph node metastases, particularly in the presence of severe postoperative scarring. The use of sonography also allows the assessment of the infiltration of blood vessels and organs, such as the thyroid gland, by adjacent nodal metastases and an accurate follow-up of patients receiving chemotherapy or radiation therapy [17].

The AJCC classification for cervical lymph nodes in head and neck cancer is not specific for the ultrasound examination. This is because some lymph nodes in the classification, such as prelaryngeal, paratracheal and upper mediastinal nodes, may not be accessible via ultrasound. In 1986, Hajek et al. established another classification of cervical lymph nodes in order to

http://dx.doi.org/10.5772/60072

simplify ultrasound examinations of the neck. According to this, the cervical lymph nodes are classified into eight regions based on their location in the neck, as shown in Figure 3 [18].

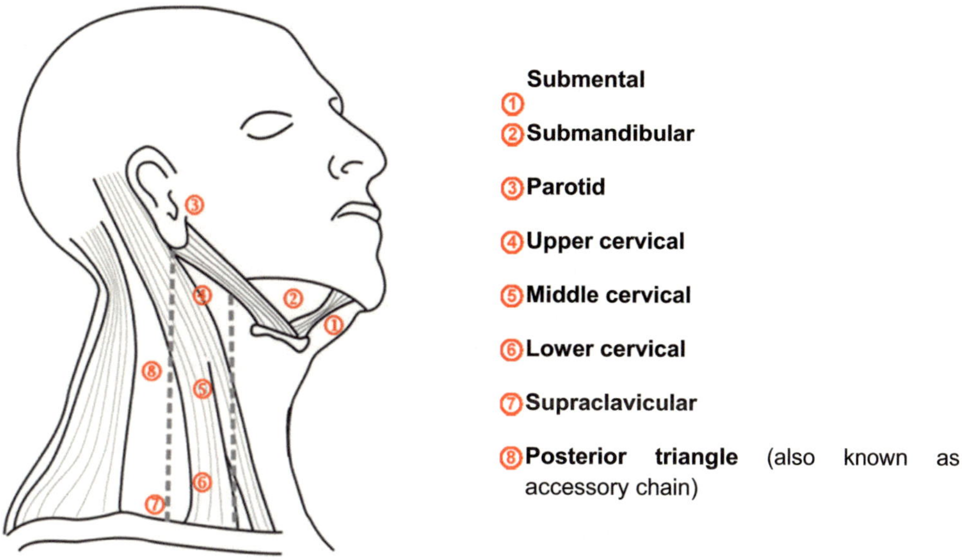

Figure 3. Classification of cervical lymph nodes for US examination [18].

In an ultrasound examination of neck lymphadenopathy, the distribution, size, shape, nodal border, echogenic hilus, intranodal necrosis and calcification are the evaluated features.

The size of normal cervical lymph nodes differs with the location in the various regions of the neck and thus, it cannot be used as an absolute criterion for the diagnosis of metastatic lymphadenopathy. The inflammatory nodes can be as large as malignant nodes, whilst a malignancy can be found in small nodes. It has been reported that the lymph nodes in the upper neck tend to be larger than those in the lower neck.

The shape of lymph nodes is usually assessed by the short axis diameter: long axis diameter (S:L ratio). A lymph node with an S:L ratio less than 0.5 is oval in shape, whereas an S:L ratio greater than or equal to 0.5 indicates round node. An oval node indicates normality, whereas malignant nodes tend to be round in shape as shown in Figure 4 and 5.

There is a difference in the border of malignant and reactive or normal nodes. The metastatic and lymphomatous nodes have sharp borders, whereas unsharp borders are seen in reactive or normal nodes. The presence of a sharp border in malignant nodes is believed to be due to the infiltrating tumour cells replacing the normal intranodal lymphoid tissue. This causes an increase in the acoustic impedance difference between the lymph nodes and surrounding tissues.

As far as the presence of hilum is concerned, the absence of it in a lymph node is a sign of metastasis or malignant lymphadenopathy, as shown in Figure 6 and 7.

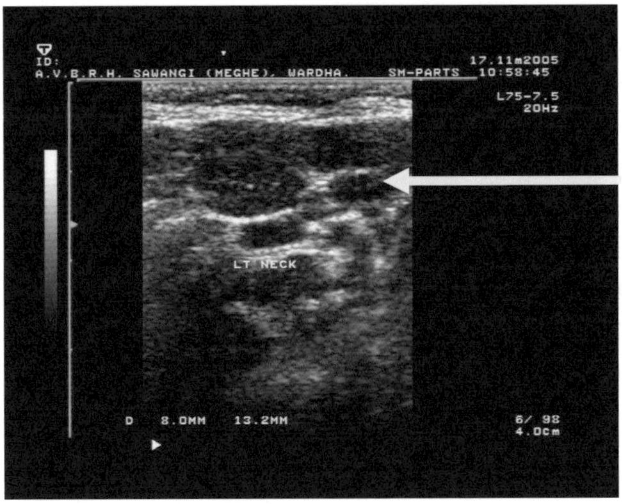

Figure 4. Sonogram showing oval reactive lymph nodes.

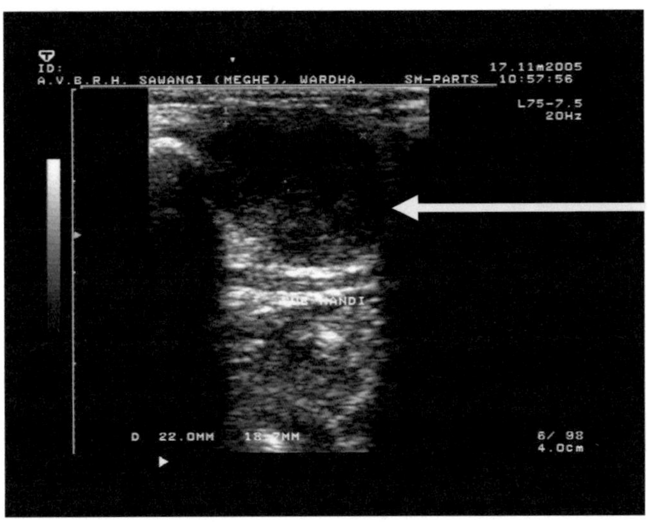

Figure 5. Sonogram showing round metastatic or malignant lymph node.

In an ultrasound examination of lymph nodes, sonologists examine intranodal necrosis and calcification. However, these examinations contribute little to the diagnosis of malignant characteristics of lymph nodes. The reason for this is that intranodal necrosis may be present in other conditions like tuberculous lymphadenopathy. Similarly, intranodal calcification also does not aid the diagnosis of malignant lymphadenopathy. This is because there are other well known causes of lymph node calcification including BCG vaccination, sarcoidosis, cat scratch disease, tuberculosis, lymphoma and fungal infections, which have been previously treated with radiation therapy.

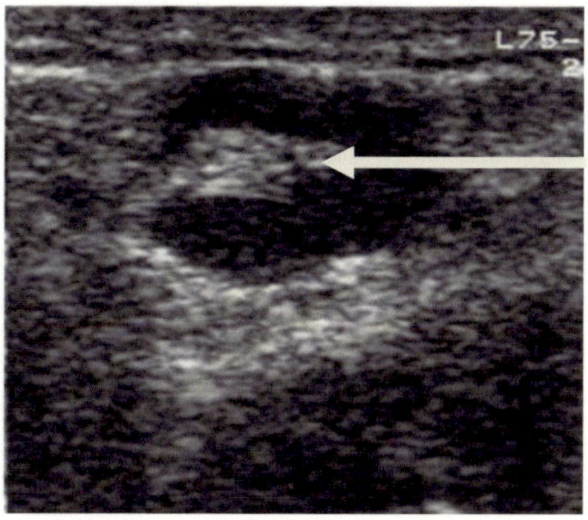

Figure 6. Sonogram depicting intact hilum suggestive of benign lymph node.

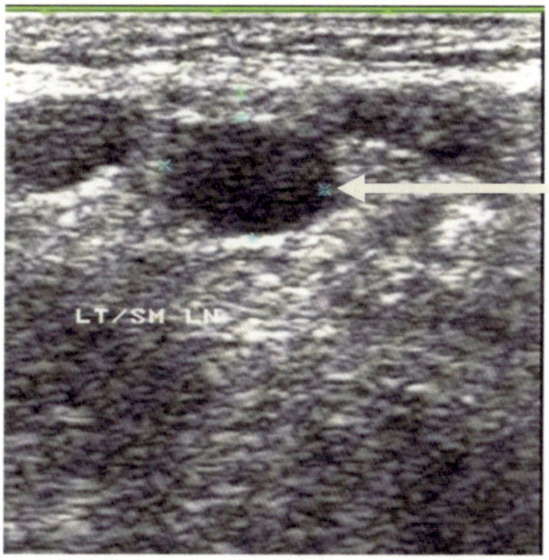

Figure 7. Sonogram showing metastatic lymph node depicting absence of hilum.

One of the advancements in ultrasonography, Colour Doppler ultrasound, can be used to define the morphologic and vascular characteristics of lymphadenopathies. Colour Doppler sonography provides information about the presence of intranodal vascularity and estimates the intravascular resistance. In Colour Doppler sonography, the pattern of vascular flow and presence of high intranodal vascular resistance have been used as key features to differentiate benign from malignant nodes.

The status of the vasculature of the lymph nodes provides additional information in the sonographic examination of cervical lymph nodes. The vascularity of the lymph node gives direction for diagnosing the cause of lymphadenopathy. This is because vascularity is directly related to the actual pathology present within the lymph node.

The characteristic event in tumour formation is angiogenesis. The morphologic and haemodynamic changes that occur in tumour vessels help to differentiate between malignant and benign lymph nodes in a Colour Doppler evaluation. In malignant or metastatic nodes, vascular structures are usually deformed due to the destruction caused by tumour infiltration and neovascularization induced by angiogenesis factor [19].

Tumour neovascularity has a particular set of characteristics. The vessels in the tumour are abnormal and show an irregular course without the progressive diminution in calibre. Furthermore, they may demonstrate arteriovenous shunting and bizarre thin walled vessels lined by tumour cells may end in amorphous spaces. The characteristic feature of tumours stimulating the growth of new vessels assists in the evaluation of metastatic nodes via Doppler sonography. The tumour vessels have a relative paucity of smooth muscle in their walls, compared to their calibre. This lack of muscular elements is reflected in the low impedance to flow, leading to a high diastolic flow and, in some tumours, the absence of systolic/diastolic flow variation [19, 20].

Both the angioarchitecture and haemodynamic differ among various cervical nodal diseases. Blood vessel morphology in metastatic nodes is usually deranged as internal nodal architecture, which is destroyed by neoplastic infiltration. Small arteries in metastatic nodes may be destroyed by tumour tissue, whereas inflammation causes the dilatation of intranodal vessels due to local humoral agents. All of these intranodal vascular alterations aid in the differentiation of malignant lymph nodes by CDUS. This is because reactive or benign nodes tend to have prominent hilar/central vascularity and metastatic or malignant nodes have peripheral or no vascularity [21]. See Figure 8 and 9.

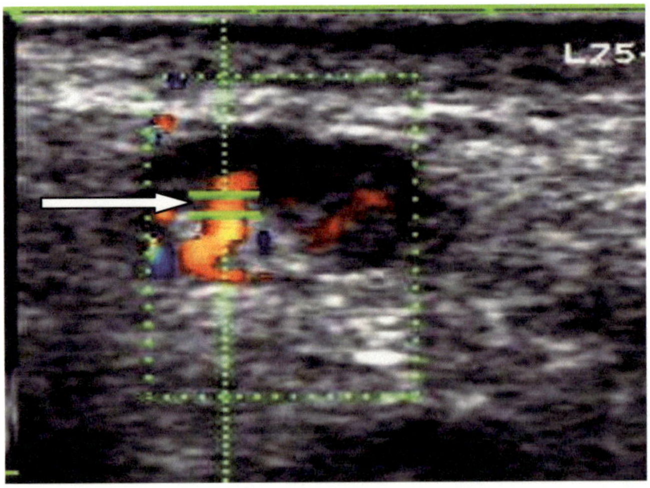

Figure 8. Color Doppler sonogram showing a lymph node with central vascular flow.

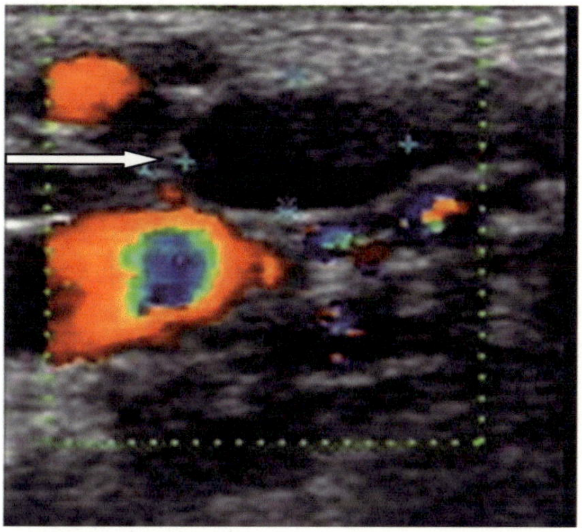

Figure 9. Color Doppler sonogram showing a lymph node with absence of vascular flow.

In advanced stages of the disease, tumour cells grow and replace a large portion of the lymph node. When the lymph node is totally replaced by the tumour cells, the tumour cells compress vessels in the lymph node. This vascular compression by the tumour cells increases vascular resistance, causing an increase in resistive index. These higher resistive indices can be observed in the metastatic/malignant lymph nodes by CDUS [21], as shown in Figure 10.

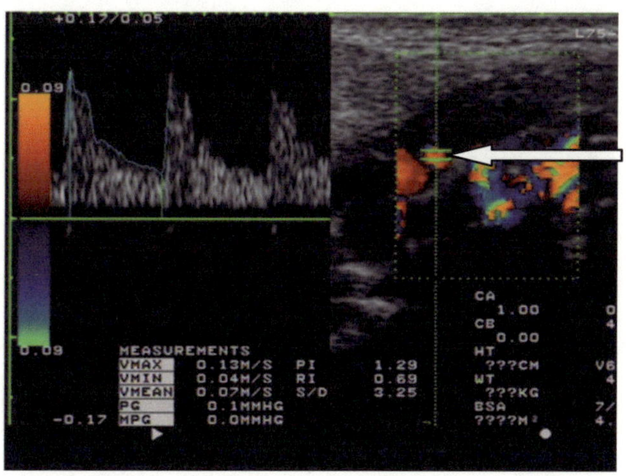

Figure 10. Colour Doppler sonogram with Doppler spectral waveform, showing a malignant cervical lymph node with peripheral Colour Doppler flow and a high resistivity index and pulsatility index.

Although Colour Doppler evaluation cannot replace the histopathological procedure in knowing the status of cervical lymphadenopathy, it plays a definite role as an adjunct to the clinical evaluation of cervical lymphadenopathy and proves its value as an important investigation [22].

5.2. Role of CT or MRI in diagnosis of local metastases in head and neck cancer

The radiographic evaluation of the status of lymph nodes is routinely performed on the basis of size, morphology, shape and margins of the nodes.

Several studies have described the radio-morphologic characteristics of lymph node metastases in computed tomography (CT) and in magnetic resonance imaging (MRI). In computed tomography, the presence of a central hypodensity in a lymph node metastasis of a squamous epithelial carcinoma is considered a sign of nodal necrosis. In magnetic resonance imaging, a central necrosis appears in the T1-weighted as a central hypointensity and in the T2-weighted image as a central hyperintensity [23].

On a CT and MRI, axial scans are usually performed. These only demonstrate the nodes in the transverse plane, where they tend to appear round or oval. Although images can be reconstructed to coronal and sagittal plane, it is time consuming and in a CT, the resolution of images is usually lower. Nodal shape does not have any value in the differentiation of reactive from malignant nodes on a CT and MRI [24].

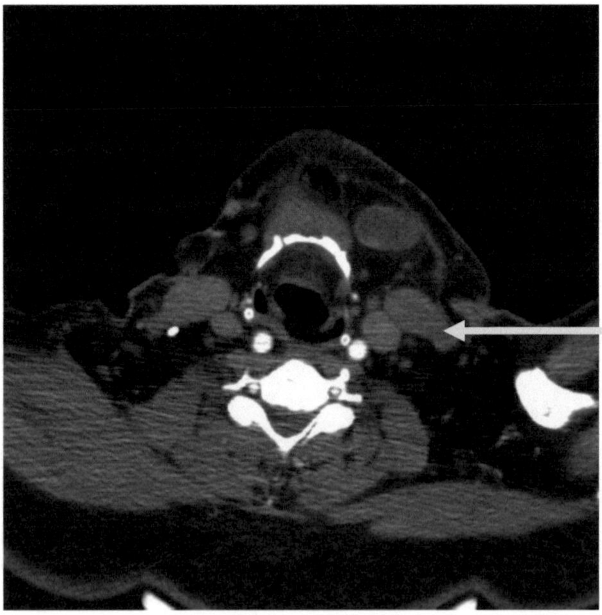

Figure 11. A CT scan of a skull with contrast reveals: homogenously enhancing lesion present in the left buccinator space, left submandibular and left jugulodigastric region lymphadenopathy. These are suggestive of a malignant lesion.

It is important to estimate the status of regional lymph nodes in cancer of any body part. In head and neck cancer, various imaging modalities should also be performed for the detection of local metastases. This is because imaging is more accurate than clinical examination. However, the assessment of nodal disease by imaging can be challenging for the radiologist. This is because there are multiple sites to review and differing opinions regarding the criteria for abnormal nodes. Hoang et al. [25] have mentioned a systematic four-step approach for the evaluation of metastatic cervical lymph nodes on cross-sectional neck imaging.

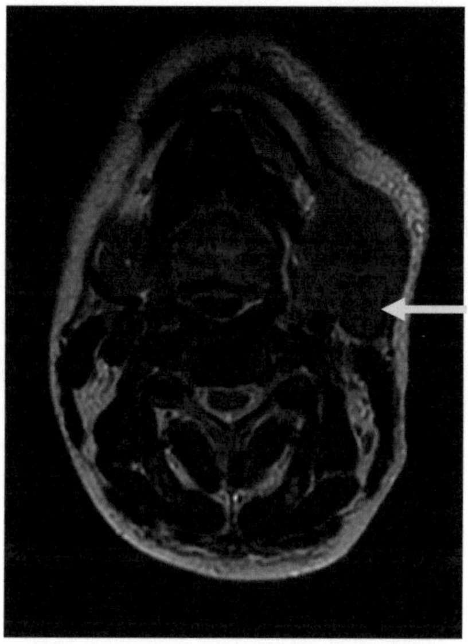

Figure 12. MRI reveals intense enhancing soft tissue mass involving gingiva, alveolus, submandibular gland and mandible suggestive of malignant lesion. It also reveals well-defined enhancing soft tissue lesion suggestive of lymphadenopathy (Axial view - T2-weighted image).

In doubtful cases of CT or MRI criteria, ultrasound is an excellent second-line tool, which can be used for evaluating these suspicious nodes and can also guide fine-needle aspiration to obtain cytology.

In oncology, the use of 18-fluorodeoxyglucose (FDG) PET has grown rapidly. This is a metabolic imaging tool that provides information beyond the anatomical constraints of conventional imaging. It can establish whether or not enlarged lymph nodes contain a tumour or are reactive. In 2005, Hain stated that PET has found more than 40% of metastases in lymph nodes smaller than 1 cm. However, the disadvantage of PET is that false positives can be found in infected nodes [26].

Kubicek et al. stated that PET and PET/CT scans have the potential to improve treatment outcomes by providing improved lymph node staging and prognostic factors [27].

Lymphoscintigraphy has been used to evaluate lymph node function. It is less invasive for delineating drainage and can help to visualize changes in the function [28].

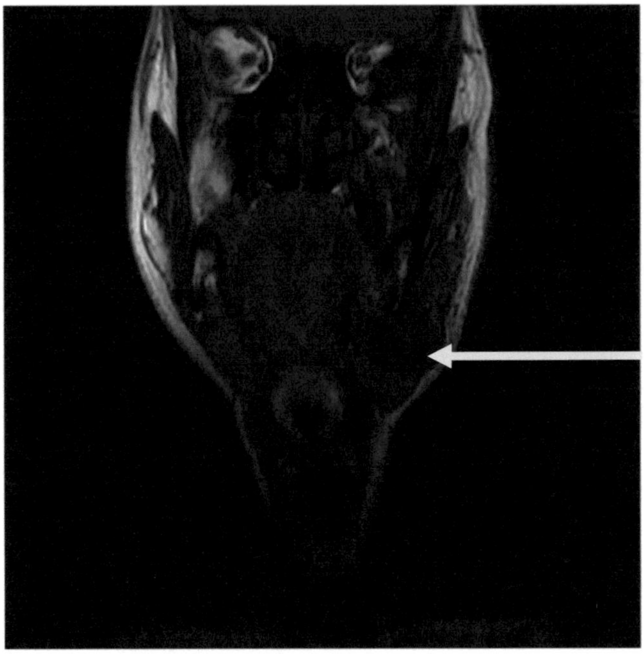

Figure 13. MRI reveals intense enhancing soft tissue mass involving gingiva, alveolus, submandibular gland and mandible, suggestive of a malignant lesion. It also reveals a well-defined enhancing soft tissue lesion, suggestive of lymphadenopathy (coronal view - T1-weighted image).

Elsewhere in the body, lymphangiography and lymphoscintigraphy are useful as these investigations provide a combination of anatomic and physiological information about lymph nodes. However, these are of no use in the neck. Both of these are invasive and can be technically difficult. MR imaging performed after the administration of superparamagnetic iron oxide particles, another hybrid of anatomic and physiological assessment, has still not been fully evaluated and is not widely available. Metabolic (functional or physiological) imaging with fluorine-18-fluorodeoxyglucose positron emission tomography is new and promising. The limited anatomic detail that positron emission tomography provides will likely require correlation with CT or MR imaging to make it widely useful.

Several studies suggested that new and highly sensitive investigations, in particular immunohistochemistry, molecular analysis, polymerase chain reaction (PCB) and serial sectioning of cervical lymph nodes, have increased the detection rate of micrometastases in head and neck cancers [29].

In addition to imaging techniques, the use of biomarkers studied on a protein, DNA or RNA level may be useful for the assessment of regional metastasis in head and neck squamous cell carcinoma [30].

FNAC and biopsy are considered confirmatory tests for the diagnosis of lymphadenopathy but these have a certain lacunae. For example, Ying et al. [18] stated in their review that it is difficult to collect adequate tissue volume from small lymph nodes and from post-irradiation nodes. According to them, it has been reported that 15% of specimens from US guided FNA did not provide an accurate diagnosis due to an uncertain diagnosis or inadequate sample. In the neck, FNA is usually difficult in a lymph node that is situated in the deep submandibular area.

Sato et al. [31] stated that puncturing the metastatic node with a needle could not be indicated in all situations because of the risks of micro dissemination of cancer cells, rupture of the capsule of the metastatic node and infection after FNAB.

6. Treatment related significance of cervical lymphadenopathy in head and neck cancer

Localized tumours that do not metastasize have the best prognosis. Cancers that have metastasized usually indicate a later stage disease and treatment becomes more complicated, with poorer outcomes. During the surgical treatment of a tumour, the nearby lymph nodes are also removed. This is because these are frequently the first sites of the cancer metastasis.

Current treatment strategies in oral cancer rely on staging based on the imaging techniques to detect regional metastasis. However, no strategies challenge the gold standard of histopathological examination of the neck dissection [32]. Nevertheless, various imaging madalities may direct the surgeons to convert the treatment plan to choose a more conservative neck dissection or, after frozen section control, to convert the treatment to a more radical dissection.

In conclusion, the presence of local metastases influences the treatment and prognosis of head and neck cancer. The traditional approach of treating all necks by considering the significant risk of having occult lymph node metastases may result in the unnecessary removal of regional lymph nodes, which ultimately prove to be pathologically free of cancer. Imaging plays a vital role in detecting the status of regional lymph nodes. For each and every patient of head and neck cancer, pretreatment imaging should be a protocol used to help to decide the appropriate treatment. Imaging performed before surgical treatment will aid in reducing mortality and morbidity.

7. Conclusion

In conclusion, the traditional approach in head neck cancer is to treat all necks by considering the significant risk of having occult lymph node metastases. Unfortunately, this approach often involves the unnecessary treatment of necks that ultimately prove to be pathologically free of cancer. So, we recommend the policy that for each and every patient of head and neck cancer, careful thorough evaluation should be performed by means of various imaging modalities. This will help to decide most appropriate treatment as well as reduce overall morbidity.

Author details

Suwarna Dangore–Khasbage

Address all correspondence to: Dangore_suwarna@redffmail.com

Oral Medicine and Radiology, SPDC, Datta Meghe Institute of Medical Sciences, Wardha, India

References

[1] Parkin D, Bray F, Ferlay J and Pisani P: Global Cancer Statistics, 2001. CA Cancer J Clin 2005; 55: 74-108.

[2] Argiris A, Karamouzis M, Raben D and Ferris R: Head and Neck Cancer. Lancet. 2008; 371: 1695-1709.

[3] Ravmond L. Warpeha. Masses in the Neck. In: Wood NK, Goaz PW (5th ed). Differential Diagnosis of Oral and Maxillofacial Lesions. St Louis, MO, Mosby-Year Book, 2005; 521-539.

[4] Okura M, Aikawa T, Sawai N, Lida S and Kogo M. Decision Analysis and Treatment Threshold in a Management for the N0 Neck of the Oral Cavity Carcinoma. Oral Oncol 2009;45: 908-911.

[5] Sheng-Po Hao, Shu-Hang NG. Magnetic Resonance Imaging Versus Clinical Palpation in Evaluating Cervical Metastasis from Head and Neck Carcinoma. Otolaryngol Head Neck Surg 2000; 123: 324-327.

[6] B. Epstein et al. Oral cancer. In: Burket's Oral Medicine. Diagnosis and Treatment, 10th edition. 2003; 194-234.

[7] Okura M, Kagamuichi H, Tominaga G, Lida S, Fukuda Y, Kogo M. Morphological Changes of Regional Lymph Node in Squamous Cell Carcinoma of the Oral Cavity. J Oral Pathol Med 2005; 34:214-219.

[8] Santin AD. Lymph Node Metastases. The Importance of the Microenvironment. Cancer 2000; 88:175-179.

[9] Mohan H. Text Book of Pathology. 5th Edition. Jaypee Brothers, Medical Publishers (P) Ltd, New Delhi. 2005; Pg. No. 442-467.

[10] Martinez-Gimeno C, Moro Rodriguez E, Navarro C, Lopez Varela C. Squamous Cell Carcinoma of the Oral Cavity: A Clinicopathologic Scoring System for Evaluating Risk of Cervical Lymph Node Metastasis. Laryngoscope 1995; 105: 728-733.

[11] Nakayama A, Ogawa A, Fukuta Y, Kudo K et al. - Relation Between Lymphatic Vessel Diameter and Clinicopathologic Parameters in Squamous Cell Carcinomas of the Oral Region. Cancer 1999; 86: 200-206.

[12] Edge SB, American Joint Committee on Cancer. AJCC Cancer Staging Manual, 7th ed. New York, NY: Springer-Verlag, 2010: 648.

[13] Greene FL, Page DL, Fleming ID, et al. American Joint Committee on Cancer. *AJCC Cancer Staging Manual*. 6th ed. New York, NY: Springer; 2002.

[14] Giovagnorio F, Caiazzo R and Avitto A. Evaluation of Vascular Patterns of Cervical Lymph Nodes with Power Doppler Sonography. Journal of Clinical Ultrasound, 1997; 25: 71-76.

[15] MacIntosh RB. Classification and Staging of Oral Cancer. Oral and Maxillo - Facial Surgery Clinics of North America 1997; 9(3): 283-296.

[16] Jonas A. Castelijns, and Michiel W. M. van den Brekel. Detection of Lymph Node Metastases in the Neck: Radiologic Criteria. AJNR 2001; 22: 3-4.

[17] Vassallo P, Wernecke KJ, Roos N and Peters PE. Differentiation of Benign from Malignant Superficial Lymphadenopathy: The Role of High-resolution US. Radiology 1992; 183: 215-220.

[18] Ying M and Ahuja A. Sonography of Neck Lymph Nodes. Part I: Normal Lymph Nodes. Clinical Radiology 2003; 58:351-358.

[19] Kenneth J.W. Taylor, Isabel Ramos, Darryl Carter, Steven S. Morse, Daniel Snower and Caren Fortune. Correlation of Doppler Ultrasound Tumor Signals with Neovascular Morphologic Features. Radiology 1988; 166: 57-62.

[20] Ahuja AT, Ying M, Yuen YH and Metrewali C. Power Doppler Sonography of Metastatic Nodes from Papillary Carcinoma of the Thyroid. Clinical Radiology 2001; 56: 284-288.

[21] Dangore-Khasbage S et al. Utility of Color Doppler Ultrasound in Evaluating the Status of Cervical Lymph Nodes in Oral Cancer. Oral Surg Oral Med Oral Pathol Oral Radiol Endod 2009;108:255-263.

[22] Dangore SB et al. Evaluation of the Efficacy of Colour Doppler Ultrasound in Diagnosis of Cervical Lymphadenopathy. Dentomaxillofacial Radiology. 2008; 37: 205-212.

[23] Maurer J, Willam C, Steinkamp HJ, Knollmann FD and Felix R. Original Investigations. Keratinization and Necrosis Morphologic Aspects of Lymphatic Metastases in Ultrasound. Investigative Radiology 1996;31: 545-549.

[24] Ahuja A and Ying M. An Overview of Neck Node Sonography. Investigative Radiology 2002; 37(6): 333-342.

[25] Hoang JK, Vanka J, Ludwig BJ and Glastonbury CM. Evaluation of Cervical Lymph Nodes in Head and Neck Cancer with CT and MRI: Tips, Traps, and a Systematic Approach. AJR 2013; 200:W17–W25.

[26] Hain SF. Positron Emission Tomography in Cancer of the Head and Neck. British Journal of Oral and Maxillofacial Surgery. 2005; 43: 1-6.

[27] Kubicek GJ, Champ C, Fogh S, Wang F, Reddy E, Intenzo C, Dusing RW, Machtay M. FDG-PET Staging and Importance of Lymph Node SUV in Head and Neck Cancer. Head & Neck Oncology 2010; 2:19.

[28] Sato T, Morita Y, Kawabata Y, Noikura T, Yamaguchi K, Sugihara K and Matsune S. Clinical Evaluation of Lymphoscintigraphy with a New Technetium Compound for Metastatic Cervical Lymphadenopathy. Dentomaxillofacial Radiology 2000; 29: 230-237.

[29] Ferlito A, Shaha AR and Rinaldo A. The Incidence of Lymph Node Micromestases in Patients Pathologically Staged No Cancer of Oral Cavity and Oropharynx. Oral Oncology, 2002; 38: 3-5.

[30] Takes RP. Staging of Neck in Patients with Head and Neck Squamous Cell Cancer: Imaging Techniques and Biomarkers. Oral Oncology 2004; 40:656-667.

[31] Sato N, Kawabe R, Fujita K and Omura S. Differential Diagnosis of Cervical Lymphadenopathy with Intranodal Color Doppler Flow Signals in Patients with Oral Squamous Cell Carcinoma. Oral Surg, Oral Med, Oral Patho, Oral Radio, Endod. 1998; 86: 482-488.

[32] Som PM. Detection of Metastasis in Cervical Lymph Nodes: CT and MR Criteria and Differential Diagnosis. Am J Roentgenol. 1992;158: 961.